Praise for John Loupos:

"Heaven and earth are embodied both ... far greater dimension than any other Tai Chi book that I've ever read, John Loupos has crafted a remarkable work. Some of my favorite sections include: 'Momentum of Your Mind', 'Ordinary Learning or Transmission', 'To Do or Not To Do?'. Here are some real tools that provide superb guidance for the serious student of Tai Chi Chuan. This is a true treasure of wisdom and grace!"

 —Mark Mincolla, Ph.D. Author of:
 The Wu Way (Pennyroyal Press 1993),
 The Tao of Ch'i (Pennyroyal Press 1995),
 Maximum Healing (Pennyroyal Press 1999)

"The ancient internal art of Tai Chi Chuan can take a lifetime to master. With the help of John Loupos' *Tai Chi Connections—Advancing Your Tai Chi Experience*, students and teachers alike will receive practical guidance on the physical, mental, and spiritual aspects of the profound art's healing and martial applications."

 —Roger Jahnke, O.M.D. Author of:
 The Healer Within (Harper San Francisco, 1999),
 The Healing Promise of Qi (Contemporary Books, 2002)

"John Loupos has dedicated his life to the mastery of Tai Chi and the Chinese martial arts. In this latest work, he offers fresh and original insights harvested along his path of ongoing study with world class masters, personal practice and teaching. Loupos takes readers on a rich and multi-layered journey that exhibits a deep sensitivity to the inner structure of Tai Chi and the deeper intricacies of releasing our old habits and beliefs so that we can open to the innate wisdom within Tai Chi training. Traditional yet radically modern, this book peels away centuries of tradition in an honest and important look at the promise and pitfalls in the classic and contemporary student-teacher relationships."

 —Jampa Mackenzie Stewart, Author of:
 The Life of Gampopa (Snow Lion, 1995)

"A good read, with many useful and insightful tips, observations, anecdotes and exercises presented in clear and down to earth language. I particularly enjoyed his discussion of the 'Congruence of Body Parts and the Mind', achievable through Taiji [Tai Chi] as a metaphor for the conduct of life itself.

 —Jan Diepersloot, Author of:
 Warriors of Stillness Vols. 1 & 2 (Center for Healing & the Arts, 1997 / 2000)

Tai Chi Connections

Tai Chi Connections

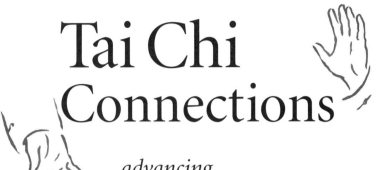

*advancing
your tai chi
experience*

John Loupos

YMAA Publication Center
Boston, Mass. USA

YMAA Publication Center
Main Office
4354 Washington Street
Boston, Massachusetts, 02131
1-800-669-8892 • www.ymaa.com • ymaa@aol.com

10 9 8 7 6 5 4 3 2 1

Editor: Eleanor Sommer
Cover Design: Vadim Goretsky
Anatomical image from LifeART, SuperAnatomy, Copyright ©1994, Lippincott Williams
& Wilkins, a Wolters Kluwer Company.

Publisher's Cataloging in Publication

Loupos, John.

Tai chi connections : advancing your tai chi experience / John
Loupos. -- 1st ed. -- Boston, Mass. : YMAA Publication Center, 2005.

p. ; cm.
Includes bibliographical references and index.
ISBN: 1-59439-032-0 (pbk.)

1. Tai chi. 2. Mind and body. 3. Self. I. Title.

GV504 .L68 2005   2005922210
613.7/148--dc22   0505

Disclaimer:
The author and publisher of this material are NOT RESPONSIBLE in any manner whatsoever for any injury which may occur through reading or following the
instructions in this manual.
The activities, physical or otherwise, described in this material may be too strenu-
ous or dangerous for some people, and the reader(s) should consult a physician
before engaging in them.

Printed in Canada

Table of Contents

Preface

When I wrote my first and then my second book on T'ai Chi, my publisher was all over my case. That is to say he encouraged me strongly to identify and narrow my audience. He felt that my books would have a more predictable appeal if they narrowed their focus to target a specific audience, i.e., beginners *or* intermediates/advanced students. I parried his advice, not because I felt the counsel was poor, but because it didn't feel right for me. As I look back, having now authored three books on the subject of T'ai Chi, I agree that yielding to my publisher's advice might actually have been quite sensible—write a book for beginners and then continue on to write progressively more advanced sequels for intermediate and advanced practitioners. The truth is, though, that I never imagined at the onset of my book writing that I would write more than one book.

It is also true that writing in a more linear fashion would not have been in keeping with the manner in which I teach T'ai Chi Ch'uan. The way I teach at my school is to maintain what I call an "entry level" T'ai Chi curriculum. This is open to all students, along with separate classes for my more experienced students. At first glance, it might appear that I do maintain some semblance of a linear hierarchy to systemize my teaching methodology. In fact, there is some linearity in the way I teach. My students do initially learn the first section of the Yang style form in the entry-level classes, with the later sections of the form generally occurring in the more advanced format.

However, the essential concepts of T'ai Chi—the essences of rooting, of structure, of energy, of living congruently—are all introduced from the get-go in my entry level classes. Students who are brand new to T'ai Chi may hear all about centerlines, or the importance of not bouncing, or how to open their *kua*, or *fa jin* power, right from the very onset of their training. Even my more experienced students know better than to skip these entry-level classes, for there is very little I deem imprudent to address in them.

My reason for teaching like this is that I believe that people "get" things when they are ready for them. If some idea or concept is beyond the grasp of certain members of my class, they may only comprehend a very small part of it during their initial exposure. But the next time they are presented with the same or some similar lesson, they will be better prepared to absorb what they weren't ready for earlier. With each subsequent exposure, progressively more pieces of the T'ai Chi puzzle fall into place. Over time, as more and more pieces fall into place; each piece serves as a reference point for the other pieces, regardless of when they appeared on the students' learning curves. In this way the "whole" of T'ai Chi begins to take shape, but only as the students, themselves, become ready for the lessons before them.

In short, my teaching method is as least as circular as it is linear, leaving me ample opportunity to customize any given lesson in accordance with students' needs. My teaching approach is underscored by my belief that if students don't get some piece of T'ai Chi the first time around, we will circle back around eventually. I have observed over the years that even the exact same lesson presented to students repeatedly, and at different points in their training, will resonate for them in progressively meaningful ways. This is because each new strata of learning allows us to adjust and readjust our perspective of the substrata that precedes it. This observation serves as a premise for my writing as well.

Just prior to completing the manuscript for this book, I had the pleasure of reading Barbara Davis's just released book, *The Taijiquan Classics: An Annotated Translation.* (Barbara is also editor of *Taijiquan Journal.*) In her book (Davis 2004, 53), Barbara notes some of the difficulties inherent in compiling credible data for a scholarly text such as hers. In particular, she notes that the *Taijiquan Classics,* which are an inventory of early and significant literary works on T'ai Chi Ch'uan espousing its most vital principles, were all written in the classical Chinese tradition. Classical Chinese, according to Barbara, "makes great use of rhythm, rhyme, poetry, alliteration, parallel prose, visual puns of written characters, aural puns based on like-sounding words, as well as allusions to or quotes from canonical works . . . (with) a tendency towards ambiguity, obliqueness, and terseness." From this she construes that "the works were not primarily intended for a popular audience." In other words, a great deal of what was written about T'ai Chi early on, and which has since come to be regarded as gospel, was intended to be comprehensible only to those already privy to T'ai Chi's secrets, or to those of a social class that could comprehend the subtleties of the written classical Chinese language. The approach of, apparently, confining T'ai Chi knowledge to members of the same "club" or social class as ascribed to by the classics is in direct contradiction to what I hope to accomplish as a T'ai Chi author. It is my intention to reveal what I can of the magic that T'ai Chi has to offer so that all readers can come away from this book both more knowledgeable about T'ai Chi and better equipped to improve their actual level of skill when practicing T'ai Chi.

Thus, I have written this book in a fashion similar to my earlier works in the belief that you, the reader/student, will glean whatever you are ready for. In all likelihood, just as is the case with the practice of T'ai Chi, subsequent readings over time will yield more meaning or further information, as you become ready for it. Happy reading.

Acknowledgements

I wish to extend my appreciation to my publisher, David Ripianzi, for his enduring support, along with that of all the staff at YMAA, especially Carol Shearer-Best and Tim Comrie. Special thanks go to my editor, Eleanor K. Sommer, and to my friend, Gretchen Sassone, whose constructive criticism has once again contributed to more lucid text. Thanks also to those students who posed for photographs; Drew, Janet, Carol, and Leslie.

I am also grateful for my many teachers and T'ai Chi colleagues and friends, all of whom have contributed in some way to my T'ai Chi experience. I have learned much over the years from my teacher and friend, Wei Lun Huang, whose influence has also inspired me to continually question and learn on my own. I would particularly like to thank my T'ai Chi teaching colleague, Lin Lin Choy, for her helpful feedback and for her assistance in enhancing the clarity of certain points by referring to original Chinese texts. My thanks go out, as well, to all those T'ai Chi students and teaching colleagues who responded to my questionnaire on teacher/student relationships (see chapter 12). Most of all, I am indebted to my many students who provide inspiration to me as both a teacher and as a writer.

Romanization of Chinese Words

This book uses the Wade-Giles romanization system of Chinese to English. There are two other systems currently in use. These are the Pinyin and the Yale systems. The cover of this book presents the Wade-Giles romanization without apostrophes in order to simplify cataloging

Some common conversions:

Wade-Giles	Pinyin	Pronunciation
Ch'i	Qi	chē
Ch'i Kung	Qigong	chē kŭng
Chin Na	Qin Na	chĭn nă
Kung Fu	Gongfu	gŏng foo
T'ai Chi Ch'uan	Taijiquan	tī jē chüén

For more information, please refer to *The People's Republic of China: Administrative Atlas*, *The Reform of the Chinese Written Language*, or a contemporary manual of style.

Prelude

Generally, the value that people attach to any educational or personal development undertaking has at least some correlation to the anticipated demands and difficulty of the task. If you expect a learning task to be difficult or laborious, you may be less likely to approach it with genuine enthusiasm. Part of my goal in writing this book is to render T'ai Chi's most exacting and intimidating aspects more easily attainable for the average student. I do this by presenting the information I have to share in clear and unambiguous prose that is easily relatable, even for beginners at T'ai Chi. In sections where I offer how-to guidance, readers will find their attempts to follow along made less complicated by clear directions. Once you see for yourself how easy it can be to improve your technique, your T'ai Chi practice will start to feel less like something you "do" and more like an indelible and joyous part of who you are.

I do want to emphasize that this book has been written as something of an addendum to my two earlier volumes on T'ai Chi. Either of my earlier books can be read and easily understood, more or less in their entirety, by T'ai Chi novices and even lay people. This should also be the case with the greater part of this text. However, this book focuses in a more detailed manner on the subtleties of T'ai Chi's mechanical aspects.

Tai Chi Connections: Advancing Your Tai Chi Experience presumes that readers have some pre-existing familiarity with T'ai Chi Ch'uan. Though readers who lack any previous background at T'ai Chi are sure to find this book engaging and informative, it has not been written with the rank novice as strongly in mind as were my earlier books. Therefore, in order for you to get the most out of this book, I recommend that you also make a point of reading either of my two previous books. *Tai Chi Connections: Advancing Your Tai Chi Experience* is just what its title implies, a deeper and more thorough investigation into structural and "real life" aspects of T'ai Chi not previously covered.

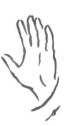

PART 1

Points to Ponder

1

CHAPTER 1

Opportunities in Slowness

"Slowness," most people would agree, is T'ai Chi Ch'uan's most conspicuous if not its most defining feature. Ask anybody to describe T'ai Chi, even someone who has never had direct exposure to this discipline, and they are almost certain to use the word "slow" somehow in their description. In fact, slowness is so associated with T'ai Chi in most people's minds that it is widely presumed to *be* T'ai Chi's defining feature. The truth is that however much T'ai Chi observers might identify or equate T'ai Chi with moving slowly, its slowness is merely a means to an end. More correctly, T'ai Chi offers up a multiplicity of ends, as there are a range of potential benefits for those who engage themselves in its regular practice.

It is T'ai Chi's slowness that facilitates the acquisition of certain of its finer and deeper qualities and associated benefits. Prominent among these are improved balance and rooting, reduced stress, and enhanced Chi (Qi) flow, as well as all the advantages and more, that one might normally expect from a nonjarring form of movement and exercise. I would add to this list the less heralded benefits of improved respiratory function, "being in the moment," enhanced critical thinking, and optimal proprioception. Surely, T'ai Chi's slowness lends it an aura of grace and beauty. But to those more practical and less aesthetically inclined critics who might ask, "What's the big deal about moving slowly?," I would suggest that were it not for T'ai Chi's slowness its full range of benefits would be less attainable. Let's take a closer look at the role slowness plays in facilitating these various qualities and benefits.

Balance

Certainly, a sense of balance is necessary for good T'ai Chi. Should you chance to observe a skilled practitioner engaged at his art, you can hardly fail to be impressed by the smooth and fluid manner in which he glides from move to move. There are moves or positions in the T'ai Chi form whereby balance seems to take priority even over rooting (to be discussed shortly), as in the moves Golden Cock Stands on One Leg, or Turn (Spin) Around and Kick. Balance is what keeps us from falling down and can usually be achieved via proprioceptive familiarity, which develops as a result of constant and regular repetition of any sought after skill. T'ai

3

Chi is hardly unique in its emphasis on balance. Other body/mind disciplines such as yoga and some forms of dance often require extraordinary balance for correct expression. However, the slow movements of T'ai Chi make the possibility of improved balance more accessible to a wider population. This includes individuals or groups for whom dance or more static yoga postures might be unsuitable, inconvenient, or less than fully adequate to their needs.

Proprioception

T'ai Chi offers the potential for a unique form of direct health benefit specifically due to its slowness and its mindfulness. By way of example, I have a student who, shortly after he enrolled for T'ai Chi classes, began to develop an awareness of certain problems with his body. As his problems persisted he sought medical council and, unfortunately, was diagnosed with multiple sclerosis (M.S.). Before you begin to wonder if T'ai Chi caused or aggravated his symptoms, I will mention that this student's wife insisted that she noted her husband's symptoms prior to his embarking on T'ai Chi, and prior to his developing any deliberate awareness of them himself. The symptoms had been there, but he hadn't paid attention to them.

Multiple sclerosis is a progressive disease characterized by degeneration of the myelin sheath that coats and insulates the nerves in the brain and spinal chord. Myelin, in addition to its protective function, increases the efficiency of nerve impulse conduction. Erosion of the myelin reduces the efficiency of conduction, resulting in symptoms typical to M.S., including numbness, tingling, muscle weakness, fatigue, slurred speech, and other symptoms, including paralysis.

Since his initial diagnosis, this student reports an overall improvement in his symptoms, even though his MRI findings indicate a worsening rather than an improvement of his condition. He informs me that even with occasional unsteadiness and numbness in his arm he has a better sense of where his body is now at any given moment than he did prior to the onset of symptoms.

So what is this account of my student's multiple sclerosis doing in a chapter on "slowness"? The slowness of T'ai Chi, it seems, facilitated an auxiliary sense of self-awareness where normal proprioceptive feedback had declined. How can this be so? Proprioception is the process by which specialized nerve receptors in the skin, joints, and muscles inform the brain about the body's relationship to its surroundings at any given moment. Normally, proprioception entails a rapid feedback loop of sorts—afferent nerve impulses inform the brain where the body is and efferent nerve impulses direct the body to enact whatever adjustments the brain deems to be in order. But with the degradation in myelin that occurs with M.S., normal proprioception can be much reduced, leaving those who suffer from this disease feeling disenfranchised from their own bodies.

In a paper entitled, "Tai Chi, a Somatic Movement Art," Bradford C. Bennett, Ph.D., a somatics educator and T'ai Chi teacher, noted that the brain processes information both proprioceptively and enteroceptively, and that the brain can prioritize one form of sensory feedback over the other, depending on its preference for first-person or third-person self-awareness. Come again? Ordinarily, a person would be aware of his hand, for example, in the third-person, i.e., "There's my hand at the end of my arm," due to the enteroceptive senses of sight, feeling, etc. Alternatively, there may be feedback from the proprioceptive receptors located in the joints, skin, and muscle spindles which tell the brain where the body is. The slowness of T'ai Chi makes it possible for the brain to be simultaneously aware of what the hand is doing objectively, as if the brain were "watching" its own hand in the more usual third-person, while at the same time being aware of the hand subjectively, in the first-person, as an inseparable component of the self. This simultaneous (or "frequently switching," as Bennett puts it) first- and third-person awareness optimizes sensory motor learning. This is significant because if there is a decline in any of the sensory feedback loops (as often happens with aging or with debilitating nervous conditions), it appears possible to develop something of a "back-up" system to compensate. It is the focus on awareness of self, made possible by T'ai Chi's slowness that allows this to happen.

In the case of my student with M.S, I speculate that though his first-person proprioception may be diminished due to myelin degeneration, the slowness of his T'ai Chi practice facilitates an enhanced "cooperation" between first-and third-person sensory awareness. In other words, even though his normal sensory feedback loops are disrupted, an auxiliary system of self-awareness is improvised by virtue of his mindful slowness. In his case, at least, this auxiliary system appears to ameliorate his otherwise debilitating symptoms.

You needn't suffer from M.S. to be a candidate for these benefits. Anyone who suffers from proprioceptive decline, such as is generally believed to occur as a "normal" part of aging process, can use the slowness of T'ai Chi to maintain or even improve proprioceptive awareness.

Rooting

For the most part, I regard balance to be a subset of rooting during T'ai Chi practice. Rooting, more so than any other aspect *is* T'ai Chi's defining quality. This is because good rooting is requisite to efficient transfer of earth force through your body. While balancing on the earth is certainly necessary for stability in certain postures, rooting requires that we *connect to* the earth. Rooting, therefore, requires more of us than merely not succumbing to the earth's gravitational forces. Rooting is what allows us to transfer force through our bodies to or from the earth in a manner that is optimally efficient. Rooting, as a T'ai Chi quality that is dynamic versus static, is most readily accomplished by applying your clear intention and concentrated attention to body/mind nuances, and adjusting yourself accordingly. Adjustments of this kind can only be learned while moving at a pace much slower than life's normal cadence.

It is one thing to be well rooted so that you are able to move force efficiently with and through your body while in a stationary posture. It is quite another to actually apply your rooting skills while maintaining a properly aligned body as you move. Because most people move their bodies more or less unconsciously—often in T'ai Chi, as well as in life—they are rarely aware of the extent to which these movements are carried by the momentum they generate. Momentum can be problematic to the extent that it influences movements in ways other than how we intend. Moving slowly, as we do in T'ai Chi, allows us to reign in our momentum and keep our movements deliberate and precise.

Stress

Stress is pandemic in modern society. Most people who feel stressed tend to attribute their stress to factors outside of themselves, as if they were somehow "stress casualties."

> **Naturally, when stress is perceived as stemming from causes outside themselves, people perceive themselves as less empowered to initiate affirmative change. The flaw in this way of thinking is that if stressors alone were responsible for causing stress then everyone who is exposed to certain stressors ought to feel similarly stressed. We know this is not so.**

People respond to stressors differently. Why? Because the great majority of the stress we perceive is a self-generated response to the world around us. Stress stems largely from people's disinclination to be truly present to themselves. Being truly present to yourself requires that you be *in* whatever moment is at hand. As simple as this may sound, most people spend the greater bulk of their time dwelling on the past and/or the future, either in reaction to what has been, or in preparation for what has yet to unfold. Offhand, this approach may appear to offer certain benefits as a strategy for successful living. But when you are stuck "out of the now," you forfeit any opportunity to influence your life in the only context that offers any real substance, the moment of now. People who live their lives inordinately out of the moment often complain that their lives feel out of control, as if their lives weren't theirs anymore. T'ai Chi may or may not effect a change in the external dynamics of your life. What T'ai Chi will do though is to slow you down, to downshift your body first, and then your mind. In this way, T'ai Chi'ers are afforded the opportunity to live their lives more in the present tense and to reclaim a feeling of being in their own driver's seat.

The slowness of T'ai Chi de-stresses us *directly* (physiologically) by redefining the demands placed on our cardiovascular system, our lymphatic system, our musculoskeletal system, our endocrine system, and our nervous system; and mitigates any tendency toward chronic sympathetic overdrive. T'ai Chi's slowness de-stresses us *indirectly* (subjectively and cognitively) by guiding us into the moment and allowing us to reprioritize the details of our personal affairs—that is, anything and everything having to do with how we perceive our lives.

Chi

Another determining factor in how our lives unfold is Chi (Qi). Each of us has Chi, or life force energy. Chi is what animates us as living beings. Yet, most people move through their lives without ever feeling or recognizing their own Chi. One reason for this is that stress causes tension in our bodies, and tension both impedes the balanced flow of Chi and precludes the quality of attention necessary to sense its subtleties. Modern life, in general, discourages this level of sensitivity. The world outside is vast and seemingly unrelenting in its demands on our attention. The Five Thieves (the five senses) are busier than ever, meaning there is ever-decreasing incentive to attend to our own internal processes.

Direct awareness of your Chi usually hinges on the quality of your attention to the world within, a world that can be every bit as comprehensive and variable as the world outside, not to mention a good deal more relevant to you on a personal level. Here, again, T'ai Chi effects us both directly and indirectly: indirectly, through its slowness, by fostering a more focused awareness of our world within; and directly by realigning our bodies in healthier and more natural ways, so that our Chi can flow though its various energy pathways unimpeded to re-establish a natural state of balance rather than one of stuckness or polarization.

Momentum

Along with a more focused awareness of the world within, momentum is another beneficiary of slowness. Actually, one of the effects of T'ai Chi is to provide us the incentive and the means to diminish reliance on shear momentum in getting from point A to wherever we need to go, whether with our minds or with our bodies. So many of the events that unfold for us—including our interpersonal relationships as they develop and evolve and even how we establish priorities and make choices—are prompted not by in-the-moment decisions that we make consciously and conscientiously, but by simple momentum. Momentum, as a cerebral dynamic, requires little conscious thought or attention.

Of course, the fact that momentum is a driving force not only in how we move our minds, but our bodies as well, is quite obvious. Tasks as simple as walking from one room to the next are usually accomplished without a second thought. How many banged knees, bruised hips, and stubbed toes can any of us attribute to our momentum while cruising along on automatic pilot during some lapse of attention?

> Momentum and mindlessness go hand in hand as co-facilitators. The slowness of T'ai Chi puts the brakes on momentum and fills the void of mindlessness with the enhanced awareness that accompanies attention and intention.

Breathing

Momentum generally precludes conscious attention to the breath. This is unfortunate because proper breathing is crucial to any cultivation, or even just maintenance, of balanced Chi. Moving our bodies slowly gives us the opportunity to breathe in the best way, that is to say fully. This, in turn, lends support to all the body's many functions, including the aforementioned balance and rooting (which lowers the center of gravity), and stress mitigation (which activates the body's parasympathetic nervous response). Slow, deep breathing also contributes to good overall fitness (which will be discussed elsewhere) because deeper and fuller breathing uses more complete lung capacity to oxygenate all of the body's tissues more efficiently.

Most people take breathing for granted and only develop good habits around breathing as a result of some insight or new interest (e.g., meditation or yoga) that encourages conscious breathing. Conscious breathing is a good habit to have. Yet, there is one potential drawback to conscious breathing in that *conscious* breathing requires your *conscious* attention. For many people the level of attention required for conscious breathing represents more work than they are prepared to commit to. Fortunately, good breathing skills need not result *only* from conscientious attention to the breath. The slow moves of T'ai Chi have a way of influencing, indeed governing, the breath when practiced over any extended study. It goes without saying that mindful awareness of all our many aspects is an important, and desirable, feature of T'ai Chi. Yet it is nice to know that even if your mind wanders a bit, proper breathing can still occur as a consequence of just moving slowly in a T'ai Chi way.

Fitness

Fitness is at the top of many people's priority lists these days. Unfortunately, most of the exercise and fitness regimes currently in vogue are either jarring on the body or unilateral to the point of detriment. I'm thinking here of contact sports, and also of noncontact activities such as racket sports, certain types of dance, aerobics, and even golf. Only a very small number of activities are both safe and balanced for all ages (yoga and swimming come to mind here), generous in the health and fitness benefits they offer, and affordable. As a nonjarring health and fitness activity, I regard T'ai Chi as foremost among these. T'ai Chi can be adequately challenging for the cardiovascular system, regardless of age. Plus, its slow rhythmic movement patterns can be effective in stimulating the body's lymphatic drainage function. T'ai Chi's slowness also makes it the activity of choice for persons who have physical limitations or who may be in various stages of convalescence. Even for somebody who is already fit and actively engaged in activities that are harder on the body, T'ai Chi can be a perfect complement, balancing body and mind.

Critical Thinking

Finally, there is a quality that allows us to fully appreciate and make the best use of all the other qualities and benefits—*critical thinking*. Aside from T'ai Chi, critical thinking occurs in some people quite naturally, and for others it can develop as a learned skill. However, the slowness of T'ai Chi fosters a different *sort* of critical thinking. T'ai Chi's slowness serves as vantage point from which critical attention can be focused inward. It stands to reason you can't think critically about something that you're not thinking about. Due to the brain's natural filtering mechanisms few people have any incentive to spend time or effort thinking about the intricacies of their body's inner workings, or of the role their mind plays (attention/intention) in influencing their body's behavior. During T'ai Chi practice your attention and intention are consciously and deliberately trained on your more internal self. One consequence of this is that your ability for self-perception becomes heightened and honed, which encourages critical thinking to occur intrapersonally. In some cases this can actually result in profound insight and accelerated leaps in personal consciousness. I, personally, can attest to having had the experience of extrasensory awareness during my practice of the T'ai Chi form. Less dramatically, T'ai Chi's slowness, and the consequent reassessment of your personal priorities, can lead to a more conscientious attunement of your own humanitarian values.

In sum, T'ai Chi's slowness may not be its most defining feature, but the opportunities that present themselves as a direct consequence of moving slowly are vast and variable, and unique to the art.

CHAPTER 2

The Benefits of Group vs. Individual Practice

"Normally, Taiji practice is a solo affair, hemmed in by the frenetic pace of daily life, [and] though Taiji is principally an individual journey, companionship along the road is to be treasured."
—Dr. Jay Dunbar from the Foreword of
Exploring Tai Chi *(Loupos 2003)*

As you might infer from the quotation above, there is no hard and fast consensus about the relative merits of group practice versus solo practice. When you practice T'ai Chi on your own *you* are the primary variable in the experience, there being no one else to take into consideration. Of course, the conditions under which you practice (e.g., terrain, lighting, weather, your most recent meal, time of day) will have some effect on any given practice session, as can other subjective aspects. But, if it's just you and your T'ai Chi, the potential for unanticipated influences from outside sources is about nil.

You are alone with yourself. It's a beautiful, brisk morning as you stroll out to your lawn, or the park, or the quiet confines of whatever personal sanctum you have available. As you stand in quiet preparation, prior to embarking on one more of an untold number of repetitions of your T'ai Chi form, you feel yourself rooting to the earth. Your body automatically enacts a multitude of minor adjustments, and your respiration softens and slows as the parasympathetic branch of your autonomic nervous system prevails, relaxing you down to a deeper level. With the first moves of your form, you feel any residual kinks in your body announcing their release and melting away. Soon your mind and spirit follow as Chi energy starts to tingle through your body's energy pathways. In the whole universe, there is only you in your oneness with all, and the timelessness of the moment you are in.

Perhaps you have been so fortunate during solo practice as to have experienced a round of T'ai Chi practice similar to that described above. Solo practice offers the opportunity to move at your own pace, and with attention to your own agenda. You can set your pace, and if you have a notion to linger over this move or that for extra practice, that's your prerogative.

Group practice, on the other hand, offers the prospect of energies mingled, whether distractive or harmonious. When you practice your T'ai Chi along with others, their presence can't help but affect your own experience. In fact, there are a number of reasons why practicing T'ai Chi in a neighborly way can yield benefits beyond what you might expect from solo training.

Whenever two or more people practice T'ai Chi together the "energy" changes. As a member of a group, you may feel an aura of anticipation, or a heightened sensitivity to the parameters of your physical space in proximity to those around you, or a peripheral awareness of timing your moves to the moves of others. Exactly how your energy changes may also depend on the specific group context. Practicing in your regular class, alongside familiar fellow students with your teacher at the helm, will likely feel different from practicing with acquaintances at the park or, in turn, with unknown peers at a tournament or T'ai Chi get-together. Regardless of the context, group practice offers you an opportunity to learn how to engage the energy of your T'ai Chi with the energy of others on a similar path.

As a teacher, I have more than the usual opportunity, incentive, and responsibility for paying attention to the dynamics of group practice. Experience has taught me that any shift in energy can be used as an opportunity to learn something new and to increase one's perceptive abilities. For example, a feeling of enhanced sensitivity and refined perception are necessary precursors to synchronized timing. Synchronized timing implies your ability to match the timing of your moves exactly to the moves of others around you. Naturally, the whole issue of synchronized timing is moot if you are practicing alone. But when practicing alongside others, each person shares equally in the responsibility for keeping the group moving in unison. (Note: In actual practice, and depending on the size of the group, if novices or beginners are involved, more experienced students might be expected to shoulder a greater share of this responsibility in order to keep the practice within the ability range of less experienced classmates.)

Synchronized timing may seem merely an aesthetic quality to casual observers, but it can take on added significance in any context in which you engage directly with others, whether in "verbal" negotiation, Push Hands practice, or actual combat/self defense. Reflect on a time when you have been engaged in a conversation or a negotiation, perhaps one that was a bit volatile, where there was a possibility of escalating conflict. Even in a relatively benign situation, short of out and out combat, the timing and nuances of your remarks, not to mention your body language, can influence how events play out. Verbal communication that is poorly crafted or ill timed can inflame versus de-escalate a situation. The sensitivity that you develop toward others, probably unconsciously, is one consequence of group practice that can help you to avoid misreads and to respond more effectively in resolving conflict before it gets out of control. By my way of thinking, group practice is clearly more conducive than is solo practice to the acquisition of enhanced sensitivity and refined perception, for the purposes of interaction with others.

From a martial perspective, the issue of timing, or synchronizing your moves to the moves of others, is especially important. T'ai Chi, as a martial art, necessarily entails interaction with others, whether for prearranged Push Hands practice or during actual combat or self-defense. Nowadays, T'ai Chi is often pursued as a personal development or fitness activity with rare thought given to its fighting application. People who opt to study T'ai Chi are often motivated to do so for reasons that are quite different from those of people who opt to study harder or more external styles of martial arts. Nevertheless, T'ai Chi can be an effective fighting system for those who train with some regard for its martial aspects. From a martial perspective, it is very important to know where your opponent is at all times and to be able to sense, instantly, if your opponent closes his distance on you. This "knowing" can stem from visually observing where your opponent is, or it can stem from "sensing" his or her proximity. Practicing with others, and developing an awareness of where they are at all times, even in the absence of a direct visual line of contact, requires a certain peripheral awareness. This is most readily developed by practicing on a regular basis in close proximately to others. Of course, merely being able to sense an opponent's approach is useless if you lack the skills to respond accordingly, but that level of ability requires preparation of a different sort.

As an aside, I would like to mention that it can be instructive for any group to vary its speed of practice. Learning how to keep your body properly adjusted while moving at variable speeds is essential from a martial perspective because, in a real situation, you may not be able to control the speed with which another person aggresses against you. Rather, you must be able to match your speed to that of your opponent. Varying the speed at which the group practices forces you to learn how to adapt to rapidly changing situations.

Another skill that group practice teaches, even if inadvertently, is how to sense and maintain a fixed distance from those around you. Though you may have never thought of this skill as such, when you practice with others, for example in a crowded classroom, the likelihood is that you naturally become aware if someone encroaches on your space. At such times you may automatically adjust the length or width of your step or stance, or perhaps the pace of your movements to allow for a more manageable distance between yourself and those sharing your practice space. The same skill, taken to a more highly developed level, is what allows you to control and maintain a safe distance between yourself and someone who poses a genuine threat.

Aside from the manner in which group practice prepares you for engaging with others in Push Hands or combat, there is simply the shear joy of sharing your time and your space with other like-minded persons who are also committed to exploring the magic that T'ai Chi has to offer. When you practice T'ai Chi, you create the potential to grow and evolve as a person. Such personal growth may not happen by quantum leaps, but every practice session leaves its mark on you in some way. Practicing en masse allows you and your fellow students the opportunity to learn from each other's mistakes and to share in each other's progress. Because there are few road maps outlining whatever route your personal T'ai Chi journey will take, group practice can offer solace in times of uncertainty and, in the words of Dr. Jay, "companionship along the way."

CHAPTER 3

Loose Ends

No qualities are more antithetical to T'ai Chi than those of stricture and rigidity. *Stricture* connotes limitation and tightness, while *rigidity* implies stiffness and an inability to yield. I admit, right off, that I made the statement in my first book that "conflict" was the quality most antithetical to T'ai Chi. But what is (a tendency toward) conflict other than stricture and rigidity personified? Whether physical, mental, emotional, or spiritual in nature, stricture and rigidity amount to little more than energetic conflict.

The opposites of stricture and rigidity are *fluidity* and *resolve*. Tacit within the concept of fluidity is adaptability, which is your ability to respond to changing circumstances. The most obvious example of fluidity and adaptability can be found in nature in the form of water. T'ai Chi is often likened, metaphorically, to water because the behavioral tendencies of the water molecule allow it to adapt to a wide range of conditions while retaining its essential and defining properties, which is very T'ai Chi-like indeed. Whether in its gaseous, liquid, or frozen state, water always remains fluid. Even the mile-thick frozen glaciers of the ice age remained fluid in their continental advance southward. As solid ice, these masses of frozen water moved fluidly, yielding, conforming, and adhering to the contours of the landscape below as they crept along, just as you want to do with your T'ai Chi.

Resolve, at first glance, has a suggestion of finality and "unrelentingness" about it, as if something were a done deal. But the finality of resolve and the stasis of rigidity are entirely different qualities. Rigidity amounts to "stuckness." Resolve is what happens when two or more forces settle into a place of relative balance. Resolve could be what happens when two individuals reach some accord. Or it could be what happens when unfathomable forces deep within the earth finally reach an equilibrium resulting in the formation of a mountain range. The whole idea of resolve is quite Daoist. Resolve, in fact, is what the Dao does or, more to the point, what the Dao is all about.

Be Fluid, Be Resolved

Getting back to what matters on a level more personal to you: we T'ai Chi'ers strive for fluidity and resolve, qualities that are most conspicuous when expressed in the movements of our form practice. When all our movements unfold with perfect or near perfect efficiency, in the absence of stiltedness or wasted energy, we achieve fluidity. When all the different and disparate parts of our bodies move in a mechanically connected (yet still fluid) manner, and without wasted effort, our bodies are in a state of resolve. Resolve implies an absence of internal conflict. Evidence of this fluidity and resolve can be observed in the flowing movements of individuals who have attained an advanced level of T'ai Chi skill, regardless of style. This, of course, should come as no surprise. Regardless of the style of T'ai Chi Ch'uan in question, practitioners who have attained fluidity and resolve possess in their T'ai Chi form the ideal venue for expressing these same qualities.

During your T'ai Chi form practice the epitome of fluid expression and resolve occurs when it is expressed *throughout* your movement, starting from the most proximal aspects of your body and then extending out to culminate at your most distal reaches. At more advanced levels of practice this quality tends to manifest, and obviously so, as a fluid looseness at the extremities. Drawing on a leg kick as an example, your suppleness might be observed extending from the hip to the knee and then outward to your foot or toes. More typically, this fluid quality will manifest from your waist to your shoulder, through your arm to your wrist, and emanate from there out to your hands and fingers, giving an appearance, if you will, of *loose ends*.

Three Reasons to Get Loose

This looseness through your wrist, hands, and fingers is significant to your practice in three ways. First, the very fact that you can manifest such a level of fluidity and resolve in your movement evidences an absence of stress and tension in your body. When and if your body is able to move freely, sans stress or tension, you will find yourself much better able to experience and express T'ai Chi's most sought after qualities.

Second, with stress and tension out of the way, you now have the means by which power can be expressed—not overt muscular power, but T'ai Chi "whipping power." Let me explain. The most effective part of a whip is its very tip. Of course, the entire length of the whip plays some role in whatever power radiates out through its tip, but the tip is the only place along the whip's entire length where full power can be discharged. Imagine for a moment that some whip-wielding person was trying to strike a whip at you, and you (not wanting to be whipped) were able to somehow move in and close the distance to block. If you could block in a way, say against the whip holder's wrist, that allowed you to interrupt the flow of force traveling along the whip's length (and avoid contact with the tip at the same time), you would effectively neutralize the whip's striking force.

Thus, the effectiveness of a whip is entirely dependent on an undeviated line of force traveling from handle to tip. Even though the wave-like force of a whip strike begins at its handle (starting with the snapping action of the wrist), the only point along the entire length of the whip where its power can be delivered with greatest effect is the tip. This is only so because the tip remains a *loose end*, despite the force passing through it. If we were to suppose that the last several inches of the whip were rigid, instead of loose, the whipping force released through the tip would be greatly reduced. In very much the same manner, you can move force through your body to be expressed whip-like through your hands and fingers. But you can only do this if your "ends" remain loose and fluid throughout.

The third benefit of fluidity and resolve manifesting as loose ends has to do with the mobilization of energy other than physical force, namely Chi, through your body. Whatever physical force we generate with our T'ai Chi is ideally augmented by Chi energy. The nature of Chi is to flow quite naturally through our bodies unless and until it encounters impediments to its natural coursing. More often than not, such impediments are self-generated. The average person's body/mind is rife with potential blockages, which can be caused by one or more factors including; stress, tension, worry, anxiety, poor diet, insufficient sleep, drugs (illicit or pharmaceutical), excess sex, and poor posture. Any or all of these can interfere with the balanced harmony and flow of Chi in your body. Lest students who have little interest in the expression of martial or aggressive force feel excluded by the topic, let me emphasize that "force," as I am discussing it here, is not necessarily aggressive or martial. Force can be of a healing nature as well, either as self-healing or for healing of others. Force, as a kind of energy in action, can even be thought of as the mechanism by which we move through life. By achieving a fluid and resolved looseness at your most distal reaches, you create the opportunity to issue or emit Chi energy or force, whether for martial or healing purposes, according to your needs at any given time.

Keep Your Mind Loose Too

The whole idea of loose ends is hardly limited to T'ai Chi's expression as a body discipline. Fluidity is something we can strive for with our minds as well. Those same virtues of fluidity and resolve that I have discussed in relation to your body can also apply to your mental state. Fluidity is something you can strive for with your thoughts and your life strategies as well as with your emotions and even your beliefs. You can begin to accomplish this fluidity through T'ai Chi practice by, first, being clear and deliberate in regard to your *attention* and your *intention*. The slowness of T'ai Chi creates an internal environment conducive to self-perusal and reprioritization. Your developing ability to shift gears, think critically, and adjust your priorities or strategies on the spur of the moment, and according to changing conditions, will all affirm that your mindset is becoming progressively more fluid as well.

Keep in mind that aspiring to a loose body is all well and good, but a loose body will be of little value to you if your mind is burdened by rigid tendencies. A mind that is open and that has a capacity for discernment and discrimination is a necessary adjunct to whatever proficiency you accomplish in freeing up your body.

> **Regardless of anything else that T'ai Chi might do for you, if, as a result of your practice, you do not feel yourself to be living your life more freely and harmoniously, you're missing a crucial piece.**

The sought after T'ai Chi skills of yielding, neutralizing, listening, responding with an appropriate amount of force, staying aligned and congruent, and so on, are every bit as applicable to your mind as to your body. Thus, it is your ability to maintain an open mind and to exercise discrimination in how you apply your skills that adds balance to the more physiologic aspects of your T'ai Chi practice. Developing a "loose ends" quality for your mental and emotional processes will help to insure that you are able to enact appropriate and effective measures in interacting with others, even in times of crisis when those same qualities would normally be least available to you.

Loose Ends Beget Loose Ends

The idea of loose ends as a tool for appropriate and effective behavior might seem most applicable in your interactions with others. However, the very act of your trying to employ "loose ends" qualities serves as a means to embody them on a deeper level within yourself. In other words, by determining to practice fluidity and resolve in your life, for example with others, you can actually become more adept at applying fluidity and resolve where it really matters: *intrapersonally*. With practice, fluidity and resolve can become more than mere techniques that you call on when you need them. They will become, instead, embedded into your deeper self as indelible aspects of who you are as a person. In this manner, T'ai Chi can help to extricate you from rigid mindset patterns and steady you on your own path of spiritual and emotional growth.

Foremost among the popularly accepted techniques for developing intrapersonal awareness are (1) sitting quietly in prayer or meditation and (2) psychotherapy. In the case of meditation, the basic idea of most meditative modalities is that you cross through a veil from conscious awareness into the realm of your subconscious, and then return with "something" (no matter that that something may be "less" or even "nothing") that leaves you better off than before. To actually accomplish this level of quietude requires a level of skill and/or patience, or even just a predisposition that may not be readily available to all people. For people not naturally inclined to the rigors of meditation, T'ai Chi may induce calm and self-awareness where meditation does not. Or, at the least, T'ai Chi may serve as a helpful co-practice to meditation.

Introspection can, similarly, occur in the context of talk therapy. Psychotherapy, like meditation, comes in many forms. Most psychotherapeutic issues probably fall well outside the bounds of severe psychopathology into what are usually classified as "lifestyle adjustment" issues. Therapy, such as is employed to address these issues, can be invaluable to the client in accomplishing some sense of personal resolve. That said, talk therapy is very often "benign," amounting, in the end, to little more than a sorting out process as the psychotherapist guides the client towards his or her own insights and realizations. Naturally, anyone suffering from mental illness or severe emotional distress is well advised to seek out the services of a qualified therapist or medical practitioner. But, for addressing more benign lifestyle adjustment issues, you may be able to accomplish much of this sorting out for yourself, given enough time and the right resources. Sadly, most of us lack the requisite time and resources to do so. Still, T'ai Chi can help you with this, either as a lone-standing discipline or, more likely, as an adjunct to counseling type therapy. At the very least, T'ai Chi can slow you down enough to help you become more self-aware.

How can you use T'ai Chi to accomplish work like this on your own? You can make some headway into your personal issues through a combination of factors: by remaining curious (that is, by keeping your mind wide open); by being flexible (avoid rigid attachments to beliefs or positions); by being nonpresumptuous (don't assume any conclusion is the answer, but see it as a basis for the next question); by being patient (talk therapy can take years, and so can self-generated insight); and by being committed to the process (no personal growth process is smooth sailing all the way).

In sum, having "loose ends" about your body and your mind is an aesthetically admirable trait as well as an indicator of certain underlying skills. Loose ends serve also as a metaphor for the quality of T'ai Chi to which you might aspire.

CHAPTER 4

T'ai Chi as a Path to Congruence & Congruence as a Path to T'ai Chi

I believe that congruence is what we all seek, deep down inside, even if we are not consciously aware of it. In a very real way, congruence, more so than peace, or happiness, or even self-realization is our holy grail. In this chapter, we will explore what congruence is and why it is so essential to our personal development. We will also look at how T'ai Chi Ch'uan can facilitate your attainment of personal congruence and how the reverse is true—that congruence can both improve your practice of and help you to live your T'ai Chi.

What Does It Mean to Be Congruent?

Living congruently means that you are able to conduct your life in such a way that all the different aspects of your self (i.e., your cognitive self, your emotional self, your spiritual self, and your physical/energetic self) exist and express themselves in ways that align with and reinforce each and all of the other aspects. As you might expect, this is more easily described than accomplished.

Congruence is a widely encompassing and not always straightforward term that can assume slightly different connotations depending on the context—physical, emotional, and so on—in which it is examined. Mostly you can think of congruence as a state of "harmony," whether it is with the people you encounter, or the environment that surrounds you, or most especially with yourself. *Resolved* is another word that comes to mind in describing congruence—to the extent that this word implies acceptance, which in turn implies an absence of conflict. Another word that may apply is *balance*, which suggests congruence when it is meant to imply a state of equilibrium, such as occurs when your body is properly aligned and rooted to the earth.

I would like to include my thoughts about the distinction between congruence and incongruence because their relative disparity is context-dependent as well. If, for example, an individual were to have a diagnosable mental illness, or even just commonplace neurotic tendencies, then what we might normally think of as incongruent behavior could be perfectly congruent within that person's psychological disposition. Strictly speaking, congruence carries no moral implication. Someone could be evil through and through and still be, technically, congruent about being evil. The same holds true for physical problems. Let us suppose that an individual has issues with an unstable knee. In this case lower back problems, though incongruent with his overall good health, might be congruent with the knee problems. Thus, it is quite possible for someone to be perfectly congruent about the manner in which he or she is incongruent. As with Yin and Yang there are no absolutes. There is always Yin within Yang and vice versa. For the purposes of this chapter, we will examine congruence in respect to its effect on the big picture of your life.

Let's Get Congruent

In my first book, *Inside Tai Chi* (Loupos 2002), I touched briefly on the role of congruence. Since writing that book, I have taken more time to ponder the relationship between congruence and T'ai Chi. Consequently, I feel that congruence is not merely complementary but, in fact, necessary to achieve one's fullest grasp of T'ai Chi Ch'uan.

My dictionary defines congruence as a sort of harmony, particularly such as might occur in geometry. This definition comes across as a bit mechanical for my tastes. I actually have in mind a much broader sense of what congruence entails. My own sense of congruence includes the part about harmony but without all the angles and arcs. I should hasten to add that getting all your angles and arcs just right is actually an indispensable part of T'ai Chi practice. For the moment, though, let us leave angles and arcs off to the side. When I ponder on harmony and congruence, I am struck by how auspicious these two words are. Both describe states of being in which there is an absence of conflict and a prevailing sense of peace and resolve. And that sounds very T'ai Chi-like to me.

In light of this, I found myself wondering, if congruence is so necessary, so valuable, and so all encompassing, then why are T'ai Chi practitioners not more obviously congruent in their practice? Being fully and always congruent is akin to being perfect. Perfection is something you may always strive for, even though you know full well that true perfection dwells beyond your grasp. The striving itself counts for something. But on the whole, congruence, like perfection, remains elusive. Even in the case of so called "evolved" individuals who may have put in years on the therapist's couch or the yoga mat or in ashrams, or walked across hot coals, or what have you, congruence is relative rather than absolute. For most people, it would seem a stretch to imagine always living our lives in perfect congruence with our selves and our environment. Congruence, thus, remains something of an ideal. Just as with the pursuit of perfection, we can perhaps takes solace in recognizing that any desire and intention to be congruent, coupled with our best efforts to be so, are at least steps in the right direction. That is to say we can at least be congruent in aspiring to congruence.

In actual practice, many T'ai Chi'ers do struggle with balance, alignment, rooting, et al. But why is it that T'ai Chi practitioners feel themselves to "struggle" at all in addressing inadequacies in their practice? I often observe students judging themselves harshly or despairing in frustration because their T'ai Chi falls below some arbitrary standard they've set for themselves. Why can't students accept that there are inadequacies to be dealt with and address those issues with the enthusiasm of any other joyous undertaking instead of regarding their efforts as a struggle? The truth is, however ironic, that many Tai Chi practitioners are simply incongruent about their quest for congruence.

Why is Congruence So Elusive?

Sadly, it is much easier, and certainly more typically human, to be incongruent than congruent. What renders our human condition so very human are our incongruities, our human frailties, and our capacity for human error. Right and wrong, good and bad, moral and immoral: these are qualities and designations that are ascribed to us as human beings alone. It is only within the context of these qualities that congruence, or its absence, becomes an issue. Our same human capacity for incongruence is rarely seen in lower life forms, especially those forms motivated in their behavior by instinct rather than by free will. In its broadest sense, the natural world is always congruent. Congruence prevails quite naturally throughout the Tao (Dao), until it bumps up against man's capacity for free will, and its byproduct—man's capacity for egocentricity.

Free will is a tenuous gift when coupled with humankind's limited scope for cause and effect, and further complicated by our tendencies toward illusions/delusions of grandeur. Our human ambitions might better serve us if we aspired to simple balance and harmony, as per the advice of the Taoist sages, rather than greatness and ego-driven immortality. It seems to me more than a little ironic that what makes us distinct from, and "superior" to other life forms is our proven ability to consistently live out of harmony with our selves and our surroundings. As self-appointed masters of our world, all indications are that we humans have chosen to steward our host planet in a way that can only bring about our eventual demise. And yet, as sentient beings, many of us do strive for congruence in our lives nevertheless. Perhaps we are not without hope.

More Impediments to Congruence

If only it were easy to accomplish congruence, everyone would be walking around healthy and well balanced; there would be no war or conflict, and mastery of T'ai Chi would be a breeze. But, of course, this is not the case. So what is it then that makes achieving congruence so challenging? We can begin to answer this question by looking to our own bodies.

As infants we start off in life more or less congruent. Adults customarily regard the bodies of very young children as awkward and undeveloped. From an adult perspective this may be true, yet a child's awkwardness and undeveloped features have little bearing on his or her congruence. When babies or toddlers move their bodies, they do so wholeheartedly, without fear, self-consciousness, or ego. The same goes for their breathing, which tends to be quite spontaneous and naturally synchronized with body movements. Thus, most children (even though they may not yet be practicing T'ai Chi) are somatically congruent, at least until they learn not to be. Before proceeding further with body congruence, join me while I shift over to the cognitive realm.

Just as is the case with young bodies, young minds are mostly congruent, until they learn to be incongruent. Miasmatic tendencies (more on this shortly) and predispositions aside, we each start life with a clean slate, *tabula rasa*. So, what happens to sabotage the congruence of youth? The extent to which youngsters develop as congruent versus incongruent is strongly influenced by the congruence, or lack thereof, of those around them—their caregivers; parents, relatives, teachers, etc., as well as their peers once they are old enough to have friends or go to school. It is when children absorb negative qualities that are beyond their abilities to process constructively (e.g., qualities such as anxiety, fear, anger, jealousy) that less congruent patterns begin to emerge in compensation for the lack of personal autonomy. Thus is learned incongruence.

Unfortunately, negative patterns often take on lives of their own as incongruence breeds further incongruence. Socialized incongruence extends far beyond childhood encounters as a pervasive influence in our society. Every aspect of modern living seems somehow to exacerbate this problem: social conformity at the expense of personal freedom, double standards, hypocrisy, racism, generalized anxiety, violence in the media, and so on. And that's just in the cognitive and psychosocial realm. Meanwhile, repetitive unilateral tasks, nutrient depleted foods, smoking, hours in front of the television or computer or behind the wheel, obesity, rampant substance abuse, pollution in all its forms, and real-life violence, *ad nauseum*, contribute in some way or another to physiological or somatic incongruence.

As if all that were not enough, latent forces from more deeply within may emerge to put the child, or adult, at odds with the world around. Each of us has forces, innate and learned, at a subconscious level that tend to prioritize their own needs, even at the expense of the greater good of our whole being. Freud identified the source of these forces as the *id*, which is comprised of amoral and/or irrational instincts whose sole ambition is gratification (the epitome of goal orientation). Along similar lines, Carl Jung identified the *shadow side*, which is made up of repressed or negative qualities that the conscious mind is unable or unwilling to acknowledge and cope with. Samuel Hahnemann, the founder of classical homeopathy, pointed out that miasms, or inherited tendencies, can pass from generation to generation to predispose the mind or the body to certain dysfunctional qualities. Thus, it seems we have a lot going against us. And indeed we do. But not so much so that we cannot exercise our free will in order to effect positive changes and growth. Lest we mistakenly regard these deeper aspects as "bad," remember that Yin and Yang are relative states of being and never absolute. Every aspect about us offers some prospect for personal growth.

The same free will that got us into trouble in the first place can also be our salvation. We may never fully recover the apparent congruence of infantile innocence. But even with our id, our shadow side, and miasms to deal with there is hope, providing we learn how to harness these aspects, or at least not do their bidding to our personal detriment. We can, with our free will, make a conscious choice to begin the steps to liberate ourselves from the constraints and negative influences that so permeate our lives. One way to do this is through our practice of T'ai Chi Ch'uan.

Why is Congruence Important to T'ai Chi?

T'ai Chi is all about congruence. Your waist and your feet and your shoulders and your hands and your knees and your breath and your field of vision must all work together with your ankles and your tailbone and your spinal alignment and keeping your *kua* open. And all those aspects must work "just so" with sinking back into your stance and then advancing forward, plus your rootedness and your *fa jin* power surges and your neutralizations. These, in turn, must both reflect and facilitate a Tai Chi frame of mind and spirit. Each of these separate parts or considerations aspires to meld beyond mere synchronization until all parts become an indispensable and inseparable component of the sum total of your T'ai Chi. Whew!

As T'ai Chi students we all make our own best efforts to "get it right." Generally, getting it right in T'ai Chi means organizing all the different components of your T'ai Chi practice into one intelligent whole, so that each part of your practice resonates with and supports every other part. We do this because T'ai Chi is very much more about being integrated than it is about being segmented and compartmentalized. As a result of becoming integrated, all the different and disparate aspects of your being are able to cooperate and function more efficiently. When your various aspects cooperate and function more efficiently, you no longer have one aspect of yourself working at cross-purposes with the others. The benefits of this intrapersonal cooperation are self evident not only in how you practice your T'ai Chi but, even more importantly, in how you live your life.

Congruence, thus, is a means by which you can derive the greatest value from your life, and at the lowest possible cost (measured in terms of undue effort, aggravation, misdirected energy, uncertainty, down time from injuries or illness, et al.). Part and parcel to its emphasis on integration, T'ai Chi is very much about economy and efficiency, which become more available as goals to be realized when you practice, or live, in a congruent manner.

The Connection Between Process and Congruence

Process, as I use the term, implies a particular kind of orientation, one that entails an attention to *how* such things as events, thoughts, feelings, and behaviors unfold. This is in contrast to a goal orientation, which concerns itself almost exclusively with end results. It should be noted that separate orientations toward process and goal are not mutually exclusive. Someone who is "process oriented" is likely to appreciate an end goal as one part of an overall process. Persons who are goal oriented, on the other hand, have less appreciation for process. Their only concern with process is the extent to which it furthers their goals. Clearly, goal orientation carries with it a narrower perspective.

As T'ai Chi practitioners, we have a vested interest in maintaining the broadest possible perspective. The open mindedness that accompanies a broader and process-oriented perspective advocates possibilities rather than impossibilities. A process-oriented perspective is likely to provide us more information overall and will influence how we make best use of that information, based not on narrow ambitions or judgmental tendencies but rather on open-minded assessments. A broader perspective also reduces the likelihood that we will be caught off guard by unforeseen circumstances because it keeps us open to a larger picture. By way of example, I am a chess player, not strong, but I play well enough as long as my perspective takes in the whole game. My downfall is that I often become careless when I sense an opponent's weakness and try to zero in for a checkmate. It is then, when I become too goal oriented and lose sight of the big picture that I inevitably succumb to some careless error. I would be a consistently stronger player if only I maintained a broader perspective. Alas, I am more committed to improving my skills at T'ai Chi, tennis, and writing than I am my skills at chess. We all have our priorities.

Admittedly, the example just provided has a tenuous link, at best, to T'ai Chi. Let me now provide an example more in keeping with T'ai Chi practice. Imagine a scenario in which two persons are engaged in Push Hands. If one pusher thinks he has an opportunity to uproot his opponent and, as a result, over invests his energy toward that goal, his attention to his own defense will be diminished. With his defense now apportioned a lower priority, he himself may be upended. Come to think of it, that does sound just like me losing at chess.

Another example of staying process oriented at T'ai Chi has to do with quelling your "inner judge," that part of yourself inclined to be overly self-critical. Quite a few of the students I have worked with over the years have displayed tendencies to hold themselves to unreasonably high or misplaced standards.

It is indeed ironic that oftentimes students who lack confidence in their ability have no shortage of confidence in their inability.

Instead of focusing on the joys of learning and small improvements along the way, these students prefer to find *dis*-comfort in everything they think they are doing wrong. This is unfortunate, and also unnecessary because sometimes even "wrong" is "right." This can certainly be the case in T'ai Chi where "investing in loss" is practically built into the discipline. A process-oriented approach can free us of the constraints heaped upon us by our inner judge. It can allow us to discern what is constructive about our practice, versus what needs more improvement—without the need to label ourselves as good or bad. What I'm advocating here is a T'ai Chi version of unconditional acceptance. When it comes to T'ai Chi, it is enough that we simply *are*.

Because congruence requires that you have all your aspects organized and cooperating it would seem that a process-oriented mindset toward your studies is more in line with encouraging this cooperation to happen. Even if you accept that a process orientation is the most advantageous approach, it will still take a lot of work for you to learn how to set aside unhelpful habits and agendas and place trust in your process as one aspect of becoming congruent. Keep in mind that because congruence is a dynamic way of being, and not just some end goal to be once achieved, it is itself a process.

What Steps Can You Take to Become More Congruent?

Now that you have a clearer sense of what congruence is all about, you are, no doubt, scratching your head and wondering how you might become more congruent in your life and in your practice. If you are already engaged in a study of T'ai Chi, the chances are that you have already taken your first steps, as evidenced by your involvement in a discipline that is naturally inclined toward mindfulness and personal process. Still, many people, even long standing students of T'ai Chi, fail to recognize that a desire to become more congruent and actually living in a manner consistent with that desire are not one and the same. I remember chuckling when a student revealed to me that he had just gotten a speeding ticket while flying along to arrive at T'ai Chi class on time. Another student I once taught was fiscally frugal to a point of rigidity. My school had an upcoming internal arts seminar that I felt would be of particular benefit to her, and which I knew she would not willingly pay to attend. When I tried, in a manner that I thought was adequately sensitive to her issues around frugality and pride, to orchestrate a scenario in which she could attend the seminar at no cost, she grew wary at first, and then outright distrustful. As her teacher, I was looking out for her long-term interests, but her prideful stuckness, and the anger it gave birth to, put an unfortunate strain on our relationship. These are but two examples of how personal incongruent behavior can work at cross-purposes with people attempting to live their T'ai Chi.

In order for you to become more globally congruent you must closely scrutinize the many aspects of your life. Clearly, this is a task beyond the scope of this book. What we can do here, though, is take a close look at how you might accomplish congruence in the context of your own T'ai Chi practice. Small improvements in congruence through your correct practice of T'ai Chi will lead to larger and more encompassing reforms. Over time, your T'ai Chi and your attention to living congruently will become mutually supporting models.

Your first goal is to become congruent about your pursuit of congruence. Toward this end, begin by committing yourself to better self-awareness and self-knowledge. After all, if you do not have the ability to see yourself at least somewhat critically and to understand yourself fairly objectively, how can you expect to recognize when shifts in your behavior or your outlook portend favorably?

How to accomplish this? The solution is simple, though it is guaranteed to require lots of hard work and diligence on your part: assume nothing. That's it. Question everything. Question your beliefs, your decisions, your motivations, your goals, and your priorities. Get involved in your own process. Most people live their lives based on assumptions and presumptions, which, by my way of thinking, is a disempowering and irresponsible way to live. Once you start questioning yourself you will be surprised at how much of your life is based on, or influenced by, unfounded premises. By "unfounded premises" I mean beliefs or understandings that you have adopted not as the result of your own sound critical thinking but because you have picked them up, mostly unconsciously, along the way from family or friends, or as social norms. What, you might be asking, has this got to do with T'ai Chi Ch'uan? Only that living presumptuously, or according to assumed or unchallenged belief systems, sets a poor stage for learning T'ai Chi, which, as we have already seen, requires an open and process-oriented mindset. To quote the famous twelfth century theologian and philosopher, Peter Abelard, "The first key to wisdom is assiduous and frequent questioning. . . . For by doubting we come to inquiry, and by inquiry we arrive at the truth."

Along with questioning yourself for deeper self-awareness, you must "show up" for your lessons, both literally and figuratively. Naturally, it will be difficult for you to make any real progress at T'ai Chi if you fail to attach a reasonable prioritization to your studies. If you can commit to a regular class attendance and/or home practice schedule, your task as a student, as well as that of your teacher whose job it is to guide you along your way, will be made easier and more predictable. Once you are actually in class, you need to bring a student's mind when you attend to your lessons. If you have concerns or anxieties from your life outside class weighing on your mind whilst you are engaged at T'ai Chi, it will be difficult for you to be fully present to yourself. This would seem a "no-brainer," but the truth is that many students arrive for class with their cup already over-flowing. You can hardly expect to make progress at your T'ai Chi if your practice amounts to but one compartmentalized experience among many.

Physical congruence at T'ai Chi is every bit as important as having a balanced outlook. Being physically congruent, however, does not mean you never make errors. Mistakes at T'ai Chi are a necessary part of the learning process—the operative word being process. Are mistakes then not the same thing as being incongruent with your T'ai Chi? Not at all. It boils down to a matter of perspective. Being in error, or making a mistake, has to do with a failure to produce desired results. Incongruence, by comparison, reflects on some flaw in the manner in which you pursue or interpret your results. You may be more or less congruent in your practice and your process, and yet still fail at reaching your goal. Congruence carries with it no guarantee of an end result.

By way of example, let us suppose that your goal is to uproot an opponent. You may be able to achieve that goal because you are bigger or more muscular despite using poor technique, or because your opponent is off balance. But this would hardly be an example of technique that is congruent with T'ai Chi principles. Where congruence is concerned, the end does not justify the means. On the other hand, if your technique is in keeping with T'ai Chi principles, yet you fail to reach your goal because your opponent's technique is more evolved, this does not necessarily reflect poorly on your own congruence. Whether or not you end up achieving your goal has little bearing on the congruence of your means.

Congruence can be one of the most challenging qualities that you aspire to as part of your T'ai Chi practice. And it can be just as challenging to maintain congruence once it has been achieved. Unlike so many other difficult-to-acquire skills, congruence can never be assumed or taken for granted. In fact, you do not "accomplish" congruence so much as you come to understand it, or even just live it, so that with each T'ai Chi practice session, and with each waking day, you set out anew to be congruent as best you can in truly living your T'ai Chi.

Concepts to Remember:
- Congruence is what we all seek.
- Congruence means your various aspects reinforce each other.
- Congruence prevails naturally in the Dao.
- We begin life naturally congruent.
- T'ai Chi is all about congruence.
- Process entails an attention to how's and why's, not just results.
- Small improvements in life and in T'ai Chi lead to more encompassing reforms.
- Assume nothing, question everything.
- Show up with a student's mind.
- Congruence carries no guarantee of end result.

In the next section, you will have the chance to apply some of this theory about congruence to your practice and to experience firsthand the benefits of getting everything working together in just the right way.

PART 2

Arranging Your Body in a T'ai Chi Way: Miscellaneous Connections

My hope is for the section that follows to be experienced by readers as a comprehensive exploration on one very important aspect of T'ai Chi Ch'uan. Any in-depth exploration of T'ai Chi could focus on its mental/emotional/spiritual component, or its energetic/Chi (Qi) cultivation component, or its technical/mechanical physical component. By my way of thinking each of these components is important to the point of being indispensable. Furthermore, none of these three is inherently more valuable, in the long run, than any other in the pursuit of a full and well-rounded development at T'ai Chi Ch'uan. However, even though these three components share equal prominence in Tai Chi's grand scheme they do not enjoy equal standing in the hierarchy of T'ai Chi skills development. One of these components takes precedence over the others.

There are any number—dozens or even hundreds—of viable paths other than T'ai Chi that anyone might follow in the pursuit of mental, emotional, and/or spiritual growth and awareness. And there must be dozens upon dozens of methods designed solely for the purpose of developing and cultivating Chi, life force energy. However, in comparison to the vast range of choices as regards these first two components, there are relatively few modalities designed so deliberately for the purpose of cultivating conscious awareness of precise technical and mechanical details and connections in your body as T'ai Chi Ch'uan. Because T'ai Chi is first and foremost a discipline characterized by movement and motion I feel its technical/mechanical aspects dictate precedence over other components in any student's scheme of learning. Emphasizing T'ai Chi's physical aspects before, but not necessarily over, its energetic or spiritual features offers the opportunity for a grounded foundation from which to then cultivate the full range of Tai's Chi's features, including its more cerebral and esoteric aspects.

CHAPTER 5

Transitions and Connections

I am motivated largely to write by my own search for truth. T'ai Chi happens to be the medium through which I conduct my search. I am also motivated by my desire to share with other T'ai Chi'ers the learnings I have gleaned along the way. This gleaning process for me has led to a better understanding of the many complex how's and why's of T'ai Chi Ch'uan. In recognition of this, one of my goals as a teacher, writer, and practitioner is to map out aspects of T'ai Chi that all too often elude critical review by students, or even teachers. I do this so that T'ai Chi's intricacies might become more available, less daunting, and less elusive for other practitioners with whom I share a common path.

I am not one to believe in coincidence. Therefore, one of my premises is that everything happens if not for a reason that is immediately evident, then at least as the effect of some cause. I believe that nothing in, of, or about T'ai Chi is random, though some of its aspects may yet remain beyond our ability to explain. Personally, I find it exciting and intriguing that we T'ai Chi practitioners can be like sleuths seeking truth both in and through our practice, and also that we can be trailblazers ferreting about for answers and understanding wherever the unexplained awaits disclosure.

In any T'ai Chi movement progression there are two considerations: the mechanical aspects of the move, and everything else about the move that is non-mechanical, namely your attention, your intention, and your Chi. In the absence of well-focused attention and clear and deliberate intention or awareness of Chi, your mechanics alone may be enough to transport you from point A to point B. Attending only to simple mechanics may be fine through your initial stages, but it is hardly sufficient to make whatever moves you've been practicing amount to bone fide T'ai Chi. Similarly, though you may be of a T'ai Chi mind, in order for your T'ai Chi to be of any real and practical value in your everyday life you must also be able to master T'ai Chi body mechanics, starting from the grosser positioning of your postures and eventually graduating to a level of nuance.

The truth is, many practitioners flail about (slowly, of course), trying to gain mastery (or thinking they already have) of T'ai Chi's subtler qualities and virtues. Qualities and virtues can be categorized as being either of the body or of the mind. Qualities of the body tend to be more quantifiable and substantial, and such qualities are linked more concretely to the aforementioned cause and effect. This is actually quite convenient because cause and effect usually entails rules, and rules make the concrete causes and effects of the body more predictably reproducible once they are fully understood.

The sections that follow address the importance and the acquisition of correct technique as it occurs in samplings of T'ai Chi transitions and body positions. In each case we will explore, in some cases in excruciating detail, the how's and why's of T'ai Chi transitions and connections as governed or influenced by certain rules and mechanics.

First a few words about rules. I do not regard these rules as hard and fast, or as particularly inventive on my part. Don't look for them to be spelled out, as in Rule #1 or the like, as they will be more or less tacit in the guidance and explanations. For the most part these rules will amount to simple expressions of applied physics having to do with body mechanics, cause and effect, and common sense. Furthermore, these rules are not meant to confine, but to serve as guidelines and frames of reference. If, in reading over any of what follows, you think you can improve on it, feel free to experiment. Experimentation worked for me.

Finally, let me disclose that not all the advice I offer here will be universally precise or, in some cases, acceptable due to stylistic differences. Different styles of T'ai Chi and different teachers have their own idiosyncratic methods of executing this move or that. Nevertheless, I stand by the great bulk of what is included in this section on the basis of the body mechanics involved. You may find that a bit of tweaking is necessary for the ensuing advice to coincide with your own or your teacher's method of practice, or even with your own body. Regardless of any minor differences, the case-by-case analyses of various moves and techniques that follow are sure to provoke thoughtful reflection on certain aspects of your practice that you may have taken for granted. By my way of thinking, nothing in T'ai Chi should be taken for granted.

There Are No Transitions in T'ai Chi

Often, the various moves of T'ai Chi are thought of as specific, easily identifiable, and clearly delineated postures: Single Whip, Snake Creeps Down, Crane Spreads Wings, and so on. This impression is reinforced by the manner in which T'ai Chi is usually depicted in the various texts—still pictures of practitioners posing in these same postures.

Between these well-known postures occur what are usually referred to as "transitions." Transitions comprise all the "stuff" that exists between postures and are the means by which we segue from one posture into the next. However, more than mere filler, transitions are every bit as essential and defining to T'ai Chi as are the more celebrated and recognizable Single Whips, et al. The truth is that there is very little difference, from the perspective of T'ai Chi essences, between the more recognizable postures and the transitions that separate them. The individual postures have particular value to the extent that they highlight certain positions for their

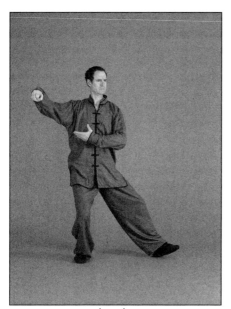

Figure 5-1 Single Whip in progress—
stepping out.

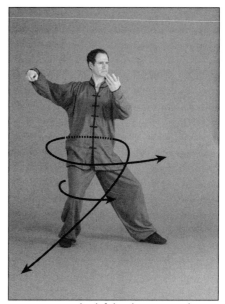

Figure 5-2 The left leg has stepped out
and the back leg now drives
the body forward.

martial application as fighting techniques or, in some cases, for physical development or for inducing energy flow within the body. Still, it is the transitions between postures that bring these techniques alive.

One way to picture this is to imagine your T'ai Chi form as a road map or communications grid map for North America. Your individual postures are like cities and towns (highlighted on the map by black dots), which are places where lots of energy tends to congregate as busyness, such as destination or departure points. The busyness of one city is only sustained in its relationship with other cities by the pathways (transportation routes and communication systems) between them. The more developed these pathways are, the better the commerce (energy exchange) is between places where energy congregates. So it is with T'ai Chi.

The fluid transfer of force and energy between postures, as well as your unerring attention to structural integrity, is what underscores the balance between T'ai Chi's softness and its tensile continuity. In the photos that follow, we can observe how the body stays connected during its transition into the move Single Whip. First we see the Single Whip in its beginning stage (Figure 5-1). Note the connections: The right knee is torqued so as to align over the right foot. Meanwhile, both the right and left *kua* are open, allowing the left knee to turn out over the left foot. Finally, the right shoulder is relaxed, facilitating a single line of force from the right wrist down through the tailbone to the earth. After stepping out with the left foot (Figure 5-2) the weight bearing right leg begins to drive the body forward, and shifts the bulk of the body's weight onto the left leg. You can see both knees are still aligned over their

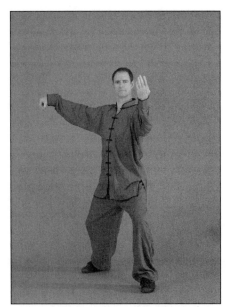

Figure 5-3a Front knee aligned over foot.

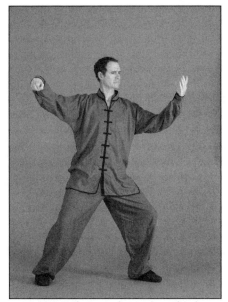

Figure 5-3b From the rear angle, the back knee is clearly aligned over its foot. Notice back foot poised to turn in.

respective feet (Figures 5-3a and b), and the right foot is poised to turn in by pivoting on its heel. The turning in of this foot will drive your right leg which, in turn, will drive force through your waist and upper body. Observe that the left palm has not turned outward prematurely. With the transition into the Single Whip posture nearly complete (Figure 5-4) observe that the right foot has turned inward. One effect of this is to straighten your back leg and torque the waist forward while you simultaneously rotate your leading palm outward (Figure 5-5).

> When you are properly engaged at T'ai Chi practice everything becomes T'ai Chi. You can see from the previous example that all the connections and details from the beginning to the end of any movement are crucial to its correct execution. There ought to be no point during your practice of the T'ai Chi form that any part of your T'ai Chi becomes any more or less representative of all that T'ai Chi is. Every movement or posture, whether it be Snake Creeps Down or Grasping the Bird's Tail, as well every part of your body—from your toes to your nose, even including those less tangible aspects of your being such as your attention and intention—can lay equal claim to non-expendability when it comes to your T'ai Chi experience.

Transitions may be the stuff that exists between postures, but postures can just as fairly be said to be the stuff that exists between transitions. Now, having established that there are no transitions in T'ai Chi, let us proceed to examine some of them more closely.

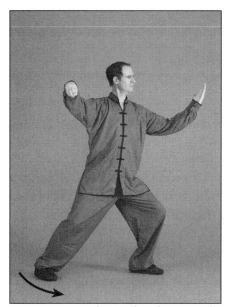

Figure 5-4 Here the Single Whip is nearly complete; note the back foot turned in.

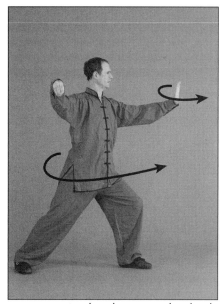

Figure 5-5 Single Whip is completed with the squaring of the waist and the lead palm turned forward.

Stylistic Differences Aside

First, prior to examining transitions, I'd like to dispel a common myth—that seemingly discrepant versions of T'ai Chi postures, as are commonly noted in comparing different styles, have any inherent aspect of being right or wrong. Different versions of the same move can often be equally correct, providing the underlying mechanics are as they should be. This simple fact can be clearly illustrated by examining several variations of the Single Whip movement noted above.

If you peruse through a cross section of T'ai Chi books, you are sure to observe depictions of practitioners demonstrating the Single Whip in variant postures such as those shown, correctly, in Figures 5-6a, 5-6b and 5-6c. In each case, the relative openness of the arms, which is the most obvious discrepancy, has little bearing on the correctness of the technique. Rather, arm angles are merely reflective of the style or teacher ascribing to that particular interpretation. In each example, the correctness of the posture is contingent on overall body mechanics rather than the aesthetics of the posture.

Now let's peruse the same three variations depicted with body mechanics in various stages of disarray. In Figure 5-7a, the subject's rear shoulder is raised. In Figure 5-7b, his chest is full rather than hollow. In Figure 5-7c, his rear shoulder appears to be correctly down, yet the exaggerated hollowness of his lower back confirms that the scapula is disconnected from the waist. In Figure 5-8a, the subject's arms are over-reaching and compromising his root. In Figure 5-8b, the right angle of the subject's rear arm to his body and waist indicates a poor scapular/waist connection. In Figure 5-8c, the subject's waist, in relation to his rear arm, has failed to

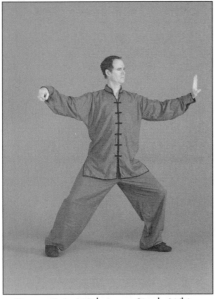

Figure 5-6a Wide open Single Whip.

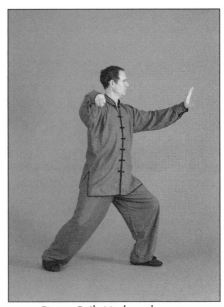

Figure 5-6b Moderately open
Single Whip.

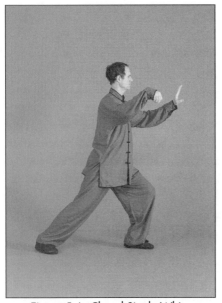

Figure 5-6c Closed Single Whip.

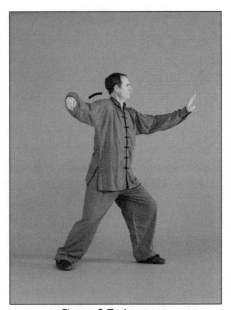

Figure 5-7a Incorrect:
Rear shoulder raised.

square properly to the front. And finally, in Figure 5-8d, the full sinking of the rear
elbow, which was entirely appropriate in Figure 5-6a, proves here to be a liability
as it undermines the shoulder/scapula connection (compare this to 5-6c).

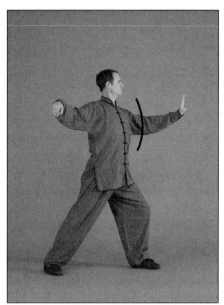

Figure 5-7b The chest is full, rather than empty.

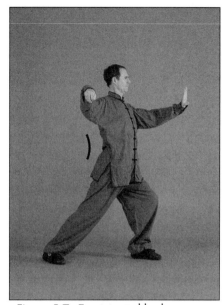

Figure 5-7c Exaggerated lumbar curvature indicates the scapula is not connected to the waist.

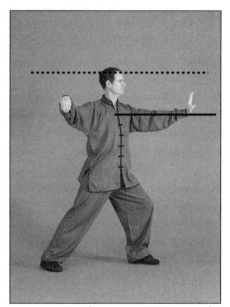

Figure 5-8a Subject's arm is overextended, causing him to bounce up.

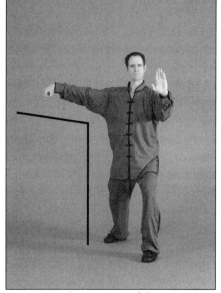

Figure 5-8b 'Linearity' of the rear arm precludes a scapular connection.

The upshot is that, regardless of stylistic differences, almost any T'ai Chi posture can be correct, providing the underlying mechanical connections have been factored into consideration. Even with a superficially "correct" overall posture, minor

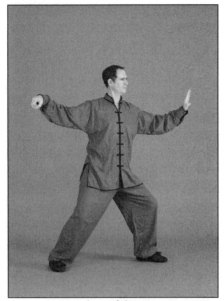

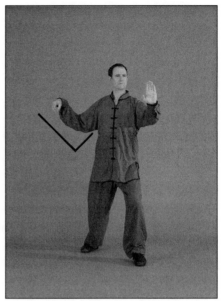

| Figure 5-8c Failure of the waist to square means the rear arm has been left adrift. | Fig 5-8d The rear elbow, overly sunk, pulls the scapula in too tight. |

discrepancies in alignment can jeopardize structural integrity at its core. Now, let's proceed to examine some of these transitions and connections more closely.

Your Initial Connection

Probably, a very appropriate place to begin our discussion on connections and transitions is at the beginning. Our first point of focus, therefore, will be on the opening move, which in most versions of the T'ai Chi form entails raising your arms and hands up in front of your body and then lowering them back down. Stylistic differences notwithstanding, if you can apply the theoretical mechanics of body structure to this first move, you will enhance your execution of it no matter what type of T'ai Chi you practice.

At either extreme, there are generally two versions of how this beginning move is typically performed. Betwixt the two extremes are any number of possible variations. In the first case there are those who lift and lower their hands nearly straight up and down along the front of the body, emphasizing the sheer verticality of the move (Figure 5-9). At the other extreme, we have those whose execution of this move has them swinging their arms upward and forward along a diagonal arc, and then lowering their arms back down in the same diagonal manner (Figure 5-10). In both cases, you can see from the arrows in the photographs that the moves appear to be, more or less, one dimensional, at least from a side view.

My preferred method of executing this move emphasizes its two dimensionality as follows. At the start of your move, press down into your Bubbling Well

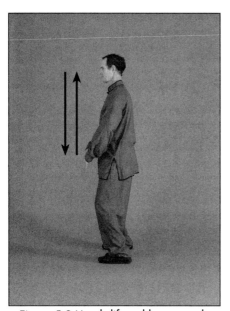

Figure 5-9 Hands lift and lower nearly vertically.

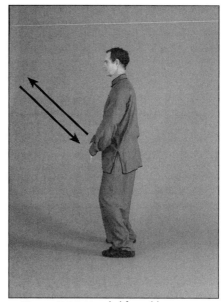

Figure 5-10 Hands lift and lower in a diagonal fashion.

point (see Glossary). As you do so, you should feel your tailbone tilt under. This may cause your centerline, from your perineum up through the middle of your body to your mid-torso, to feel as if it is lifting a bit. Any such lifting sensation comes from your *kua* and from opening your back, but the lifting sensation should feel well short of raising your body in any way that compromises your root (Figures 5-11a and b). For more detailed information, reference *Exploring Tai Chi* (Loupos 2003, 83-86), where I discuss the concept of rising up without bouncing. Next, while taking care to keep your arms properly engaged (by relaxing the scapulae open and without lifting your shoulders), begin to swing your arms forward and upward. As your arms begin to rise up, shift your tailbone from its tilted-under position to slightly tilted out to the back. This will help drive your arms forward with a structural impetus (Figure 5-12).

As your arms and hands reach up and out, approaching their furthest extension from the body, begin to curl your tailbone under again (Figure 5-13). In consequence to this curling under of your tailbone, feel your elbows "set" as your wrists and hands "round out" at their farthest extension point (Figure 5-14). At this point, you should feel as if your tailbone is connected to your elbows, and from there to your arms and hands, by ropes and pulleys.

Continue to lower your arms as shown (Figure 5-15). As your arms settle back down to their lowest position, prepare to repeat this sequence by, once again, pressing into your Bubbling Well point and articulating your tailbone under. Figure 5-16 depicts the movement sequence in it entirety. Notice that despite the "lifting,"

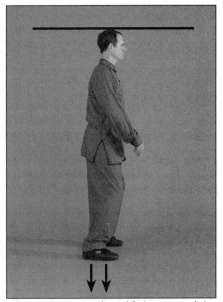

Figure 5-11a Ready to lift the arms while pressing down into feet.

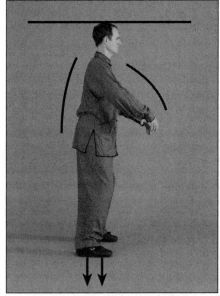

Figure 5-11b As the arms lift, feel the body open and fill, but without bouncing up.

or rippling, of the middle body due to the articulation of the tailbone, the head does not bounce up. Practice this over and over until it feels natural.

Of course, it is perfectly acceptable for you to modify the advice given to coincide with your own preferred method of practice. You may also find it helpful to exaggerate the tilting of your tailbone when you first practice this movement. As you improve your grasp of this through continued practice, you will be able to gradually tone down the range of movement of your tailbone (without forfeiting any of your mechanical advantage) to a point where the movement is barely perceptible.

Please note that this two dimensional figure 8 concept (Figures 5-17 and 5-18) is applicable to either of the two

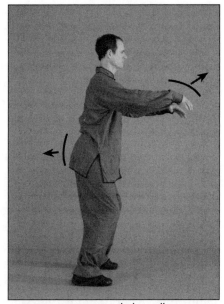

Figure 5-12 Next, tilt the tailbone out while raising the arms forward.

initial examples of the initial Tai Chi move. No matter how linear something may appear to be in T'ai Chi, you can always maneuver your body in such a way as to capitalize on the potential of a figure 8 (spiraling) energy pattern.

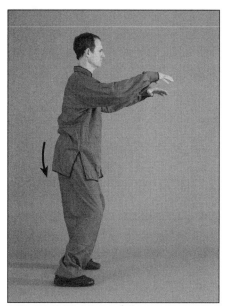

Figure 5-13 Prior to full extension with arms curl the tailbone under.

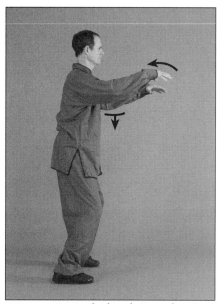

Figure 5-14 As the hands "round out" at fullest extension, the elbows set.

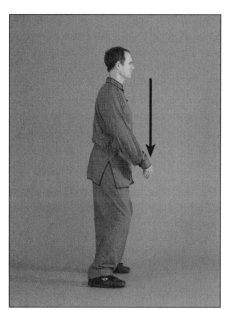

Figure 5-15 Hands and arms recovered to starting position and prepared to repeat.

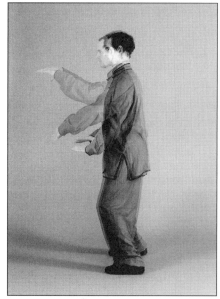

Figure 5-16 The sequence in its entirety.

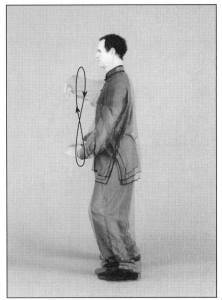

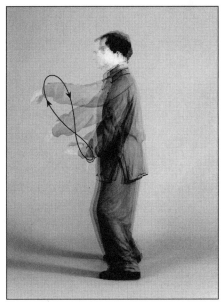

Figure 5-17 Figure 8 energy within a "vertical" movement . . .

Figure 5-18 . . .or in a more diagonal version.

Your Guy-Wire Connection

A recurring theme for many practitioners is the challenge of keeping yourself reliably rooted, or even just balanced, as you transition from posture to posture during form practice. One very helpful technique for developing a firm "rootedness" is to visualize parts of your body as having (or even as being) guy wires extending down to the earth. *Guy wires,* if you are not familiar with the term, are those stabilizing cables that can be seen anchoring and securing high wire towers or circus tents to prevent them from being toppled over by wind.

During your practice of the T'ai Chi form, you will have many opportunities to apply this visualization with excellent results. Elsewhere in my writings, I have disparaged that bane of all T'ai Chi practitioners: bouncing up during your practice to the detriment of your root (Loupos 2003, 81-89). By employing this guy wire visualization during form practice, you should be able to mitigate, if not eliminate, any tendency you have toward bouncing during your transitions. An example of how to use your guy wire imagery can be seen in the following description.

Begin by positioning yourself in a right-foot-forward Brush Knee posture (Figure 5-19). Prepare to step forward into a left-side Brush Knee by sinking your weight from your forward, right leg back onto your left leg (Figure 5-20). Then, turn your forward (right) foot outward and along with it your waist and upper body (Figure 5-21). This is the point where many students, as they begin to shift their weight onto their forward legs, are prone to losing their roots. Bouncing often occurs either as students shift their weight forward (Figure 5-22), or after they shift

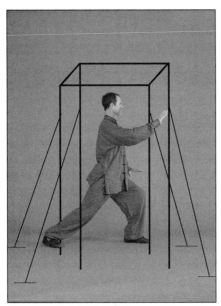

Figure 5-19 Brush Knee posture.

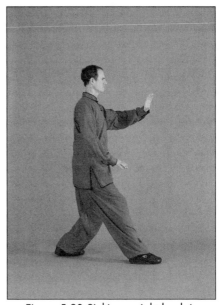

Figure 5-20 Sinking weight back in preparation to turn.

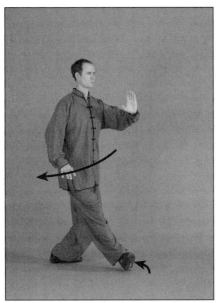

Figure 5-21 Right foot, waist, and upper body all turn right as the weight begins to shift forward.

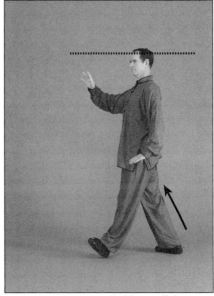

Figure 5-22 Incorrectly lifting off the root in shifting forward (From left. Note straightened back leg).

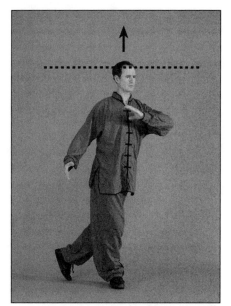

Figure 5-23 An example of bouncing off the root after shifting forward (note straightened front leg).

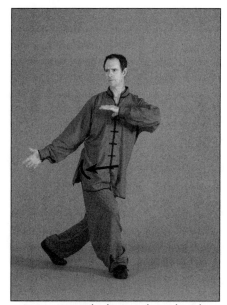

Figure 5-24 The kua on the right side is collapsed.

and as they begin to lift their back legs and feet, prior to actually stepping through (Figure 5-23). The most common cause of bouncing during this transition is an inadequately opened *kua* (in this case on your right side) due to some weakness in the supporting leg (Figure 5-24). Usually, but not always, bouncing at this juncture is accompanied by a posture that is somehow tilted off its central alignment (Figure 5-25).

You can avoid this tendency to bounce, or tilt, as you shift your weight forward by imagining that your right arm extends down and connects to the ground just like a guy wire anchoring a circus tent (Figure 5-26). Maintain this feeling of a guy wire connecting you down to the earth until you have managed to plant your front foot (Figures 5-

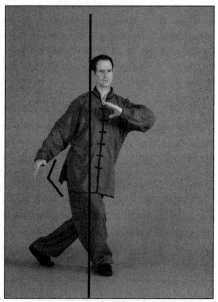

Figure 5-25 Centerline has been compromised by a protruding tailbone and a tilted head.

27a, b, and c). During this transition you can also derive benefit toward keeping your alignment centered by imagining a second guy wire attaching from your

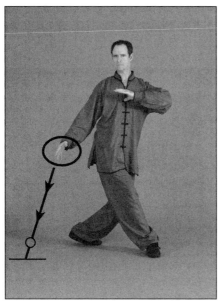

Figure 5-26 Right arm acts like
a guy wire.

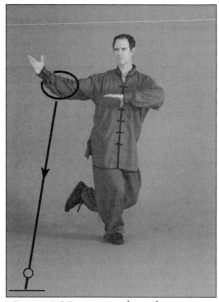

Figure 5-27a Arrows shows how to use
the arm as a guy wire while
stepping up . . . ,

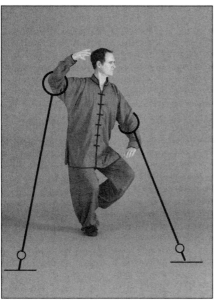

Figure 5-27b . . . stepping through,
and . . .

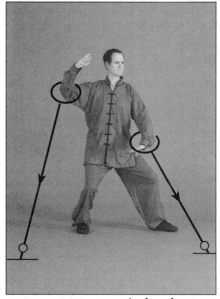

Figure 5-27c . . . as the front foot is
placed down.

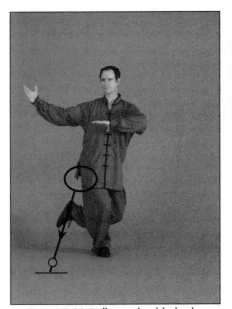

Figure 5-28 Tailbone should also be anchored with a guy wire.

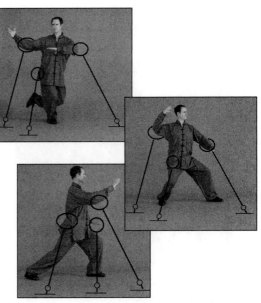

Figure 5-29 Guy wire(s) can constantly readjust as the body repositions.

tailbone and stabilizing its connection to the ground below (Figure 5-28). As your Brush Knee move unfolds, so will the positions of your arms. And as your arms shift, so should the imagined guy wire attachment points from your body down to the earth (Figure 5-29). Throughout your move, try to maintain a constant feeling that your guy wire is connected from your tailbone downward.

In the same manner that you have imagined guy wires stabilizing your body during the Brush Knee move, you can apply this model to other moves as you see fit. This visualization is especially helpful during Push Hands, or anywhere else in your T'ai Chi where better rooting is called for.

Follow the Money

There is an oft used and predictable line that one often hears in who-done-it movies. Whilst lesser sleuths are scrambling about following up on what inevitably prove to be the wrong clues, the hero detective always picks just the right moment to advise "Follow the money." How true! In movieland, and often in real life, the money trail is sure to lead you to the real perpetrator. You need look no further than the most recent corporate or political scandals for evidence of this truth.

One would hardly think that such a sordid truism could be applied to the learning of T'ai Chi. Well it can't. But I see an analogy. If we substitute the word *force* for *money*, voila! we now have some very good T'ai Chi advice indeed.

In the same way that the hero detective was able to follow the thread of financial shenanigans, deal by deal and invoice by invoice in order to get to the heart of the matter, a Tai Chi practitioner who follows the "force" will be similarly enlightened. In T'ai Chi you may express force from any given point in your body, usually from some extremity such as your palm or fore-arm or elbow. But that force must have originated from somewhere else. Just as less insightful detectives tend to get side-tracked following the wrong clues, students newer to T'ai Chi often unwittingly misplace the full focus of their attention on whatever part of the body they are using to discharge their force. They give little heed to how or where that force was generated in the first place. Consequently, these students are never fully in control of their force. If they are not fully in control of their force that means their force is in control of them. This is bad. Why? Because, at best, an inefficient expression

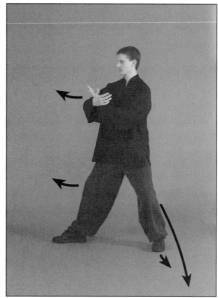

Figure 5-30 Starting from a pre-Press posture the knees are just slightly flexed with a solid earth connection.

of force is wasteful. At worst it can result in serious injury, and I don't mean to your opponent. The most likely scenario is that consistently poorly expressed force will gradually result in chronic imbalances in your musculature and/or skeletal frame. These will, in turn, spawn other imbalances until some part of your body either breaks down or experiences pain. Your training will suffer, to say the least.

Not to worry though. Problems such as these can be avoided and an efficient use of force can be accomplished by simply tracing force to source. You can follow your force in reverse, like a sleuth, along its path of travel or, better yet, from its source forward. Because your force, at any given point, is premised on the force behind it, starting from the source of your force will likely be more expeditious than working backward. Of course, this line of thinking runs counter to that of our hero detective. It presumes you know who embezzled your funds from the get go, but hey, that's a happy difference between Tai Chi and high finance.

Let's utilize the move Press as a basis for our exploration of force. Start examining from your earth connection to make certain that your feet are firmly ground-ed (Figure 5-30). Have a partner check each of your knees in turn, with each leg positioned as it would be just prior to your point of fullest extension into your Press. Your partner should be able to feel a continuum of force and stability at each checkpoint as you proceed from there to complete your move (Figures 5-31a and b). Assuming your partner did not reveal any flaws (Figure 5-31c and d) in your technique, you can move up to your next point(s).

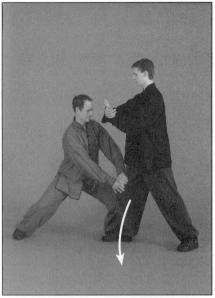

Figure 5-31a A partner checking the front knee connection . . .

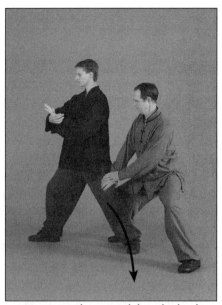

Figure 5-31b . . . and then the back knee connection.

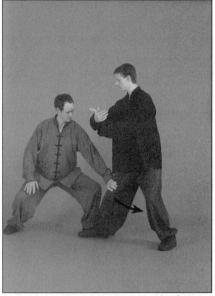

Figure 5-31c Incorrect: Here the front knee is shown turned in with a flawed connection.

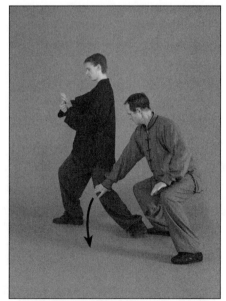

Figure 5-31d Incorrect: Here the back knee is shown buckling under a flawed connection.

Have your partner shift his attention to the checkpoint(s) at your waist/hip area (Figure 5-32a and b) in order to check for a continuum of power through your waist. Do the same at your abdomen, chest, shoulders, and arms (Figures 5-33a

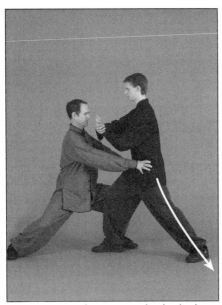

Figure 5-32a The partner checks the hips connections.

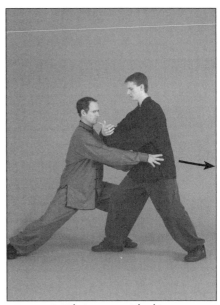

Figure 5-32b Incorrect: The hip connection fails under duress.

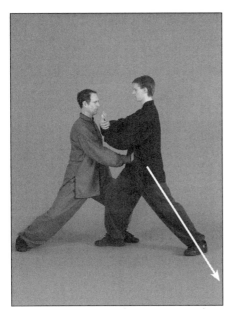

Figure 5-33a A good connection at the abdomen.

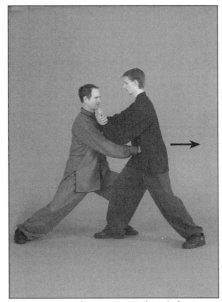

Figure 5-33b Incorrect: The abdomen connection fails to hold.

and b, 5-34a and b, 5-35a and b, and 5-36a and b). In this way, you can check to insure that there is an efficient and uninterrupted line of force coursing all the way from the earth out to your discharge point. Using this method to determine an

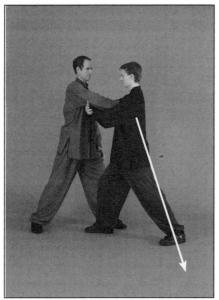

Figure 5-34a A good connection at the chest.

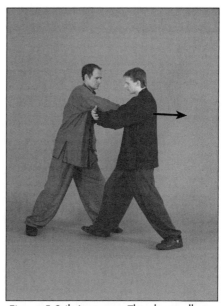

Figure 5-34b Incorrect: The chest collapses under duress.

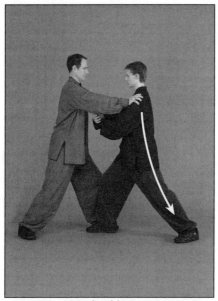

Figure 5-35a Shoulders must connect with everything below.

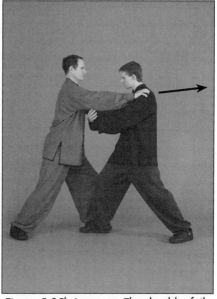

Figure 5-35b Incorrect: The shoulder fails to connect.

uninterrupted line of force from source to point of expression may not be as glamorous as "following the money," but it is a reliable means of insuring that your body stays properly connected throughout any given move.

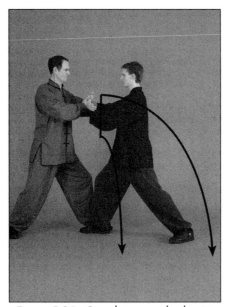

Figure 5-36a Complete your checkpoint review at the Press point.

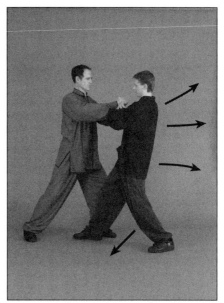

Figure 5-36b Incorrect: Weakness at Press point undermines the whole technique.

Wave Hands Like Clouds, But You Still Gotta Step Right

The move known as Wave Hands Like Clouds is one of T'ai Chi's most beautiful and recognizable sequences. Just as there are different versions and styles of T'ai Chi Ch'uan, so are there numerous ways of interpreting the role of the arms in this particular pattern: small circles, big circles, close in, or extended away from the body. Cloud Hands, as it is often called, can be downright hypnotic to the casual observer. Almost universally, the primary focus of attention while watching, or even practicing, this move falls on the hands and arms which are, after all, waving. Small wonder.

What I would ask you to pay attention to here, though, is not the hands, but the *footwork* that accompanies this pattern. In particular, pay attention to the foot with which you step out. I've heard some debate about the correct way to step during Cloud Hands, regarding which part of the stepping foot, exactly, touches down to the ground first, and this has prompted a good deal of reflection on the matter. What I have concluded is that there are three acceptable variations for determining precisely how you step. Some people step out with the toes extended and touch the toes down first and then the heel. Other folks step out to touch with the heel first, setting the foot down heel to toe. And some practitioners prefer to reach out to touch the whole flat of the foot down at once.

Stepping with the toes first seems to me the easiest of the three variations in terms of the demands on your body (Figure 5-37). The extension or depth of your supporting leg, which depends on the relative straightness or degree of flex at the

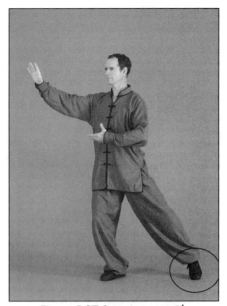

Figure 5-37 Stepping out with
the toes first.

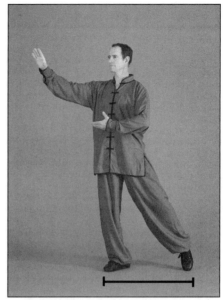

Figure 5-38a Here the supporting stance
is higher, so the toes step closer.

knee, can easily be adjusted according to your personal ability and the strength of your leg muscles (Figures 5-38a and b). Stepping with the heel first (Figure 5-39) is my preferred method of practice as it places more of a challenge on the supporting leg to flex at the knee and to coordinate that flex with the waist and the tailbone. Stepping out with the flat of your foot (Figure 5-40) strikes me as the most difficult variation because it challenges the supporting leg to sink more deeply, even beyond that of stepping with the heel, plus it places a demand not found in the other two variations on your hip abductor muscles. In addition, stepping out with your foot flat requires extra care that you not collapse your *kua* in front or tilt your tailbone out to the back (Figures 5-41a and b).

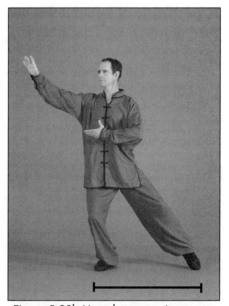

Figure 5-38b Here the supporting stance
is lower, so the toes extend out farther.

With three variations to choose from, which of these methods is the best? After experimenting with each of the various options, I am of the opinion that no one

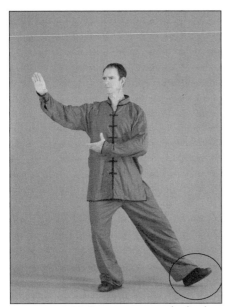

Figure 5-39 Stepping out so the heel touches first.

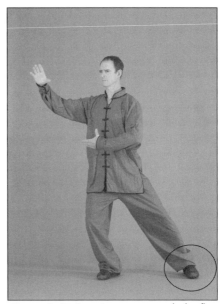

Figure 5-40 Stepping out to touch the flat of the foot down first.

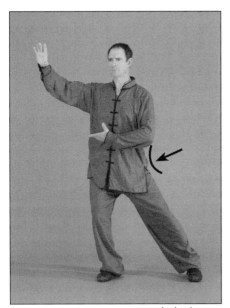

Figure 5-41a Front view with the kua collapsed inward.

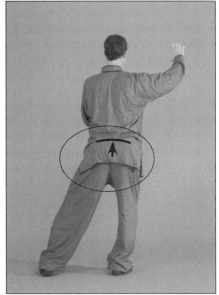

Figure 5-41b Rear view with the tailbone tilted out to the back.

method is inherently better than any of the others. That is not to say these various methods are all the same, nor is it to say that they are casually interchangeable. On the contrary, each of these three methods of stepping offers different advantages

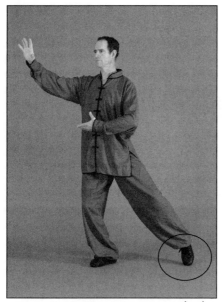

Figure 5-42a Stepping out toes to heel.

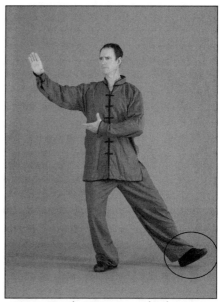

Figure 5-42b Stepping out heel to toes.

and requires separate consideration. As long as you pay heed to these considerations, however, one method of stepping is as serviceable as another.

The important point for you to keep in mind is that the correctness of your stepping technique, regardless of which approach you opt for, cannot be fully assessed until and unless it is viewed in the larger context of how your waist and upper body are positioned while you are stepping. The suitability of any of these stepping variations can only be determined in its relationship to the rest of your body. If you turn your attention to the series of photographs that follow (Figures 5-42a, 5-42b, and 5-42c), I will guide you through several considerations that typically escape the untrained eye. Let's start with a quick look at each of

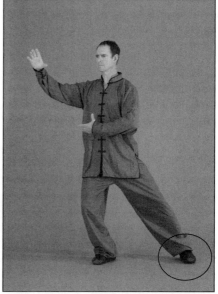

Figure 5-42c Stepping out with the flat of the foot.

these three options: in Figure 5-42a, the subject is stepping toe to heel; in Figure 5-42b, the subject is leading with his heel first; and in Figure 5-42c, our subject is

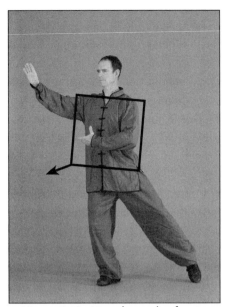

Figure 5-43a Note the angle of waist rotation in the next three photos. First, the body is turned slightly away from the stepping direction.

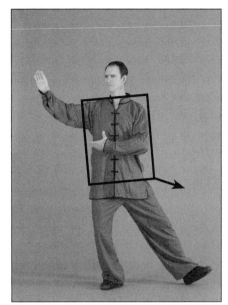

5-43b Next, the body is turned slightly toward the stepping direction.

placing his foot out flat. Notice that in all three cases the subject's opposite arm and hand are extended, which act in part as a counter-balance for the stepping foot. Ostensibly, these are very similar looking photos, with the foot positions being the only obvious differences.

However, if you look more closely at each of the photos, you will notice that there are several other discrepancies. First, and most important, each stepping variation shows the subject's entire upper body, including his waist, torso, and chest, at a slightly different degree of rotation (Figures 5-43a, 5-43b, and 5-43c). And, at first glance the angle of the supporting leg—the line from the hip through the knee to the foot below

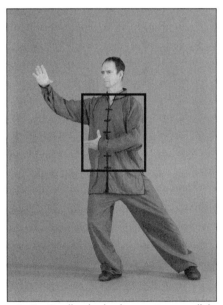

5-43c Finally, the body remains parallel to the stepping direction.

(Figures 5-44a, 5-44b, and 5-44c)—is not readily apparent, but is made more so by the overlaid graphics. Finally, though nearly impossible to discern from the frontal perspective of the photos, is the position of our subject's tailbone relative to the rest

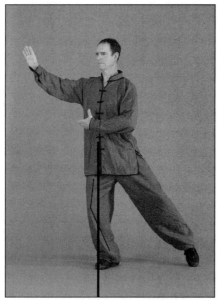
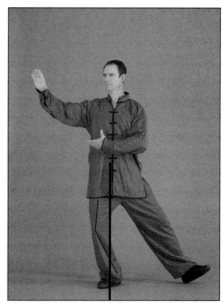

Figures 5-44a and 5-44b The three photos on this page highlight the subtle, but significant variations in the angle of the supporting leg, hip to knee to ankle.

of his body. Even so, the position of the tailbone can be inferred from the position of the hip and *kua* (Figures 5-45a, 5-45b, and 5-45c). In each case the body is aligned slightly differently. Yet, in each case the different alignments are not wrong; they are merely different. Each alignment remains fully congruent with the principles of structure.

We see that there are at least several different ways that the stepping out part of Cloud Hands can be performed. Yet simply acknowledging this does little to help you understand how or why the variation you opt for can be practiced in a way that renders it fully compatible with T'ai Chi principles. What then is the significance of these slight variations in positioning, and what concerns ought

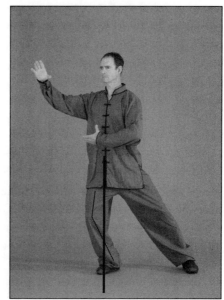

Figure 5-44c

you to bear in mind during your practice of this move?

Whenever you step *forward* in T'ai Chi, regardless of the move, in order for your stepping foot to become weight bearing, such as in Ward Off, you must place

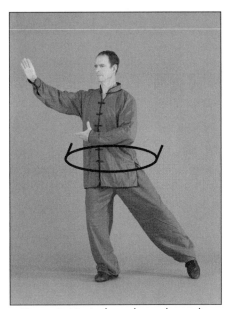

Figure 5-45a In these three photos the seeming discrepancies in body positioning are made acceptable by correct orientation of the waist and tailbone. Here the tailbone is facing toward the stepping direction (back).

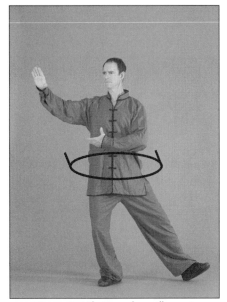

Figure 5-45b Here the tailbone is facing away from the stepping direction (forward).

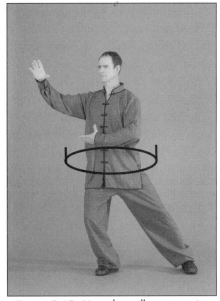

Figure 5-45c Here the tailbone remains perpendicular to the stepping direction.

your heel down to the ground first. Only then may you place the rest of your foot down flat. (The exception to this rule is when your back foot takes only a half step forward, as in Playing the Lute.) Otherwise, you would find yourself falling forward with momentum into your stance, instead of stepping forward with balance. Conversely, if rather than advancing forward, you were stepping *backward* (retreating), as in Repulse Monkey, you would need to touch the toe part of your foot down first for the very same reason, to ensure that you step, not fall.

Therefore, the part of your foot that must touch down first during Wave Hands Like Clouds sequence is determined by whether you are stepping forward or backward relative to the position of your waist and upper body. If you refer to any of the Figures, 5-42a, 5-43a, 5-44a, or 5-45a, you will see that the subject, according to his degree of waist rotation, is actually

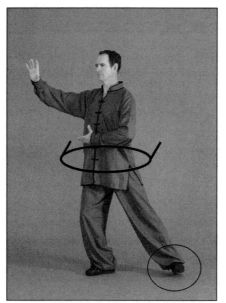

Figure 5-46a Touching the heel down first, which is incongruent with the body position.

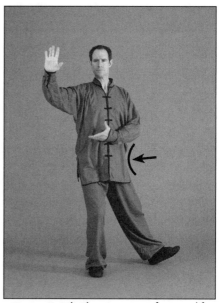

Figure 5-46b The same step from a different angle, where you can see how the supporting kua has collapsed.

stepping more backward than forward. Therefore, he is, correctly, reaching with his toes. Meanwhile, the subject in Figures 5-42b, 5-43b, 5-44b, or 5-45b has his waist rotated more toward the direction of his step, so that he needs to extend out with his heel first. It is both possible and acceptable when stepping out with your heel first to align your waist forward (away from the direction of the step) just as you might if you were stepping with your toe first. But, in order for this variation to be structurally viable you must still turn your waist into the direction of your step prior to committing your weight onto the stepping foot. Alternatively, stepping out with the flat of your foot requires that you step at a perpendicular, to the side, as seen in the Figures 5-42c, 5-43c, 5-44c, or 5-45c. In this case, your waist and upper body position must be neutral, leaning neither forward nor backward.

If, hypothetically, you were to ignore the correlation between the direction in which your waist is rotated and that part of your stepping foot that you touch down with first, your body's positioning and structure would be misaligned. For example, in Figure 5-46a, the subject's heel is reaching to touch down first, which is incorrect because his waist is turned away from the step. In this case, the direction of his waist forces him to commit his weight onto his stepping foot prematurely. Consequently, he is unable to maintain structure in the *kua* on his supporting side (Figure 5-46b). Next, in Figure 5-47a, the opposite error is shown. The subject is stepping toe first whilst his waist is turned forward in the direction of the step. The flaw in this step will not be evident until he tries to put his foot down flat (Figure 5-47b), at which point his waist and *kua* will be vulnerable to

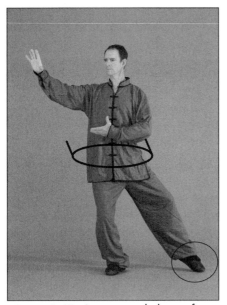

Figure 5-47a Stepping with the toe first.

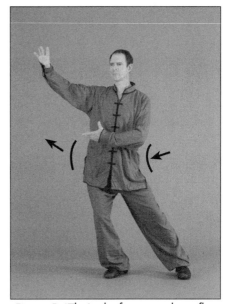

Figure 5-47b As the foot goes down flat, the waist and the kua on the stepping side collapse.

collapse just as they were in the earlier example. Ideally, however you choose to step, you will need to maintain structure throughout your transition.

Whichever of these stepping variations you opt for is up to you or your teacher. As I mentioned earlier, I have my own personal preference. But even with my preferred method, I still take care to practice all three of these methods so that I don't become locked into one way or another. I encourage my students to do the same. As long as your step correctly reflects the positioning of the rest of your body, you should reap the benefits of the movement.

Your Knee: Turn It or Torque It?

It is often the case during T'ai Chi

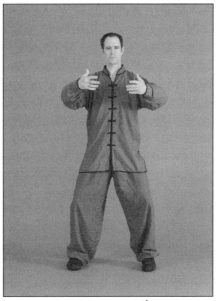

Figure 5-48 Basic Wu Chi stance.

practice that even the smallest and most discreet articulations can effect major changes in how your body connects or fails to connect down to the earth. One such example can be seen in the basic T'ai Chi posture, the opening stance, or Wu Chi

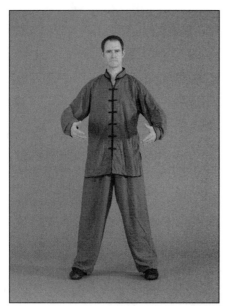 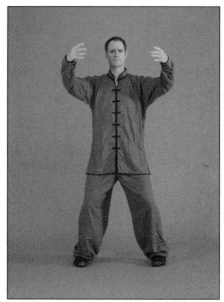

Figures 5-49a or b Standing meditation positions.

posture (Figure 5-48). The particular articulation I'd like to review has to do with how you go about positioning your knees as you stand upright in preparation to begin your form. Though this particular posture occurs infrequently over the course of the form, the principles of knee positioning have a broad application spanning the whole of your T'ai Chi form. The advice that follows will be of special relevance, as well, to any readers who rely on simple upright postures as a basis for standing meditation (Figures 5-49a or b).

It is fairly common knowledge among T'ai Chi players that their knees should be positioned slightly outward in the opening posture so as to align over their feet. The question I raise here is—should your knees be "turned" outward, or should they be "torqued" outward? The issue of turning versus torquing is not simply one of semantics, nor is this question merely academic. Your knees are a critical juncture point in connecting, or rooting, the whole of your body down to the earth, so getting this right is quite important.

Let's start by examining the distinction between these two variations: turning and torquing. The visually observable differences are subtle enough that they are unlikely to draw your attention unless you are looking closely for them. To establish a baseline, let's begin by referring to the first photo (Figure 5-50), in which you can see an individual standing with his legs completely straight. Note that the outsides of our subject's feet are aligned parallel as well. In order for the advice that follows to be applicable for you, your feet will also need to be positioned parallel. At this point, you can observe that our subject has not yet committed to positioning his knees as they have neither been flexed nor have they been turned or torqued outward over his feet.

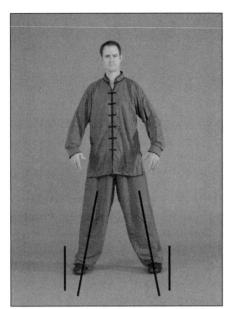

Figure 5-50 Standing straight. The reference lines show that the knees are not yet aligned over the feet. Short lines show the outsides of both feet to be parallel.

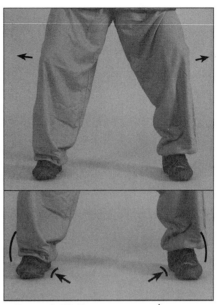

Figure 5-51 Knees are turned out over the feet. Lower photo shows insteps peeled up in.

In the next photo (Figure 5-51), our subject has "turned" his knees outward. Look closely at the inset photo to observe that the subject's insteps have peeled up slightly from the earth, causing his weight to shift laterally from being centered over his feet to now being positioned over the outer edges of both feet. The lifting of his insteps, alone, is sufficient to cause a loss of root. Additionally, turning his knees in a way that peels up his insteps places an unhealthy stress both on the ankles and at the outside of both knee joints. And, wait, there's more: "Turning" the knees also causes the tailbone to tilt outward (to the back) in a manner that exaggerates the lumbar lordosis and compresses the lower spine while filling the chest (Figure 5-52). You get all this just from "turning" your knees outward.

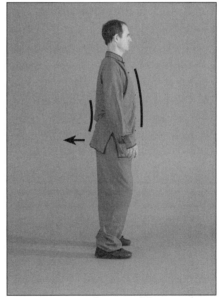

Figure 5-52 Side view of the previous photo reveals that the tailbone is tilted out and the lower back compressed in.

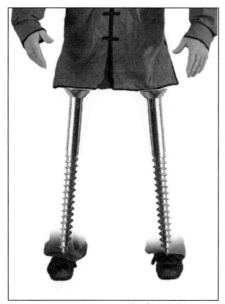

Figure 5-53 Imagining the lower legs as giant screws.

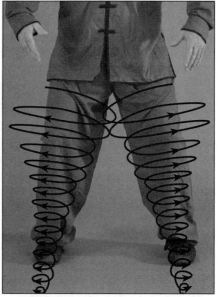

Figure 5-54 The screw threads and arrows indicate the direction of turn to tighten the legs down.

Now, let's compare "turning" against the alternative of "torquing" your knees out. First, imagine that your lower legs are like screws (Figure 5-53). Your right leg has threads that will tighten down to the earth by rotating clockwise, while your left leg is exactly opposite, requiring a counterclockwise rotation in order to tighten down (Figure 5-54). Stay with me now. Because the imaginary threads on your screws are widely spaced, like those on sheet metal screws as opposed to machine screws, only a very small degree of rotation will be required to drive each screw into the earth and, thus, anchor your legs and feet firmly down to the earth as well. Try to torque each of your screws (knees) outward by a small twist of five degrees or so, just until your knees

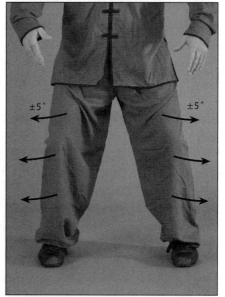

Figure 5-55 A small degree of rotation positions the knees over the feet.

are directly over your feet (Figure 5-55). You will feel that the effect of torquing fastens your feet more firmly flat to the earth.

The imagery of torquing your knees outward is uniquely applicable to your

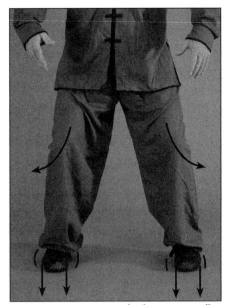

Figure 5-56 Torquing the knees out pulls the feet more firmly down to the earth.

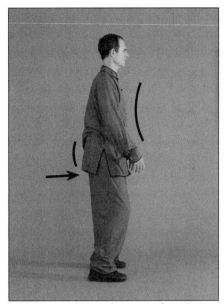

Figure 5-57 The side view confirms that torquing curls the tailbone under, decompresses the lower spine, and hollows the chest.

T'ai Chi. Implicit in the torquing of each screw is the idea that your feet will become more firmly attached to the earth—in essence, screwed down to the earth (Figure 5-56)—rather than less firmly attached as was the case earlier with turning example. You will also notice that torquing does not create the same stress at your ankles or knees as does turning. Furthermore, torquing your knees will draw your tailbone in and under, the effect of which will be to open and de-compress your lower spine and allow the chest to hollow (Figure 5-57).

Of course, it makes sense to bear this distinction in mind whenever you place yourself in the Wu Chi standing posture. This posture provides an ideal context for examining how to adjust and align your knees. Remember, though, that torquing, rather than simply turning, either or both of your knees outward is an adjustment you can experiment with in nearly every posture in your form.

A Shortcut That Makes Sense: The T'ai Chi Punch

Shortcuts can be a mixed blessing. Sometimes they work out for the best, and other times not. If a shortcut backfires, it can end up being more labor or time intensive than the original course of action you might have taken. Shortcuts can also be activity dependent. For example, in psychotherapy shortcuts may very well prove counterproductive. This is because a results-oriented approach often interferes with the growth and insight that, by design, stem from the therapeutic process. The same might be said of certain artistic or creative endeavors for which efficiency and expediency is not the primary goal. Indeed, there are certain aspects of T'ai Chi that do not lend themselves to shortcuts—aspects where the opportunity for deeper comprehension and mastery would be undermined were they not allowed to evolve on their own, uninterrupted, over time.

Still, shortcuts can be enormously valuable when they save time and effort or when they streamline efficiency. The shortcut that follows ought to be of genuine value for any T'ai Chi practitioner not already privy to its mechanism.

I was prompted in this particular lesson by a long-time friend and teaching colleague, whom I encountered at a T'ai Chi training camp. This woman is someone whom I hold in high regard for her grasp of T'ai Chi as a heart and soul discipline. Yet, despite her many years of practice at T'ai Chi, she lacked a thorough grasp of T'ai Chi's application as a martial art. She lived her T'ai Chi behaviorally, by which I mean in apparent congruence with T'ai Chi's essential principles. But her grasp of T'ai Chi as a "living discipline" did not always reflect itself in the way she moved her body structurally. This absence of structural congruence is a dynamic not uncommon in the T'ai Chi world, where the focus on fighting and even fighting theory is not always paramount. In short, this woman was not a fighter, and this was a fact that reflected itself too obviously in the way she practiced the movement part of her T'ai Chi.

As it happened, she and I were practicing in close proximity one afternoon when I noticed that her punching technique, during the move Parry and Punch, was anything but connected. Whilst her left leg/foot was forward, she was issuing a right-sided punch that drooped and then looped from her right thigh outward about a foot wide of her waist before finally ending up extended out to the front. Ironically, her punch ended up exactly where it was supposed to end up (Figures 5-58a and b). If anybody had been checking for correct positioning just at the conclusion of the technique, her punch would have earned a passing grade. This, however, was one example of the end not justifying the means. That her punch finished in the correct position hardly mitigated the fact that her delivery had rendered her punch totally ineffective. The wide swinging arc of her right arm meant that she had little more than the momentum of her fist as a power source, meager at best when you consider the relative size and weight of a fist.

What this woman was missing was a continuity of power traveling from the earth (where practically all power can be traced from) through to her fist as her designated point of contact. She had no clear sense of bringing power from the earth up to her waist for the transfer via her elbow to her fist. Instead, she was opting for the long route: up her back, around her shoulder, and down her arm, which was a misdirection of force.

In this woman's case, a shortcut was definitely called for. In order for her to deliver an effective punching technique, in accordance with T'ai Chi principles, she needed to change the delivery of her punch in a way that allowed her to move force more efficiently from the earth to her fist. She needed to reroute her power by adjusting the way force moved through her body's "power receptacle" areas,

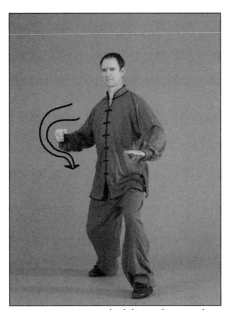

Figure 5-58a Punch delivered too wide.

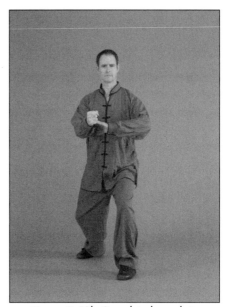

Figure 5-58b Completed punch in correct position.

specifically her waist and right elbow. A lack of continuity of power is a common problem for many practitioners, especially for those without a pre-existing foundation in more martially oriented styles. Unless you train with regard to practical application, there is little reason or incentive to emphasize the development of aspects such as optimally efficient power transfers. Yet, the types of body connections fostered by training with attention to martial applications are essential to good T'ai Chi, even if you have no desire to become a fighter.

The simplest way to accomplish this particular connection is to start by positioning the inside of your elbow directly against your waist (Figures 5-59a and b). Imagine that your elbow is attached rigidly, as if by hardware, to your waist and tailbone. To test that you have this connection, ask a partner to lean, gingerly at first, against your fist from the front (Figure 5-60). Assuming your connection is solid, very little effort will be required to withstand your partner's push, and you will feel his force traveling down through your body to the earth (Figure 5-61) instead of lodging in your arm and shoulder.

Before proceeding, let me offer a cautionary note. As a rule, closing your armpit, as will likely happen when you bring your elbow into your waist, is ill advised in T'ai Chi. Therefore, your elbow-touching-against-the-waist connection, as described here, is only temporary, until you can replicate the same quality of connection with the elbow positioned away from your body. If, while positioning your elbow against your waist, you are able to keep your armpit somewhat open (Figure 5-62) by all means do so.

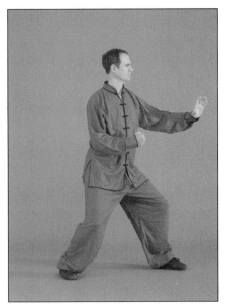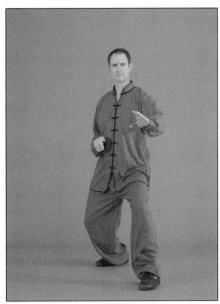

Figures 5-59a and b Start by positioning the elbow against the waist.

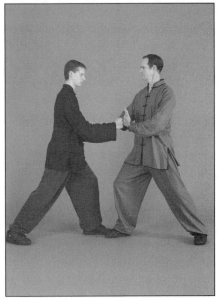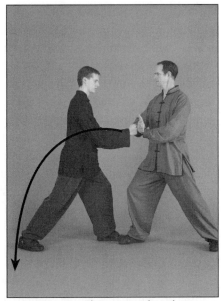

Figure 5-60 Testing the connection by having a partner lean into the fist.

Figure 5-61 The arrows show how a partner's force should redirect down to the earth.

Once you have accomplished this feeling of connection, you can begin to reset your elbow's starting position progressively farther back along your waist. Practice resetting, an inch or two at a time, until the contact point of your arm against your

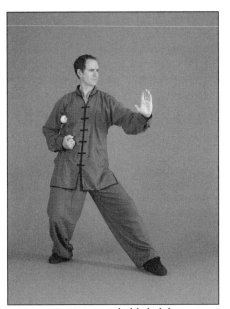

Figure 5-62 Armpit held slightly open, even with the elbow against the waist (note tennis ball as spacer).

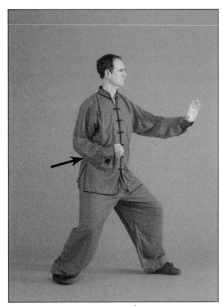

Figure 5-63 Reposition the contact point from the elbow to the forearm.

waist falls about two thirds of the way down the inside of your forearm (Figure 5-63). Be careful though, because drawing your elbow back too far will cause your shoulder to lift and weaken its connection at the scapula (Figures 5-64a and b). With this in mind, try to keep your shoulder relaxed and settled down, working on this connection until it feels natural.

Even closer scrutiny, as this adjustment to your technique comes to feel more familiar, will reveal the role of your lower body in this technique. Once your right leg has driven your body forward (Figure 5-65), your left (opposite) leg plays a prominent role in driving force through your waist in order to power your right fist forward. (Figure 5-66).

For now, though, let's keep it simple and not get ahead of ourselves. First, try to develop a familiarity with the feeling of this connection by maintaining a physical contact between the inside of your right elbow and your waist, as shown in Figures 5-59a and b. Eventually, you will shift this contact to your forearm once you have learned the elbow part of this technique. As mentioned earlier, you should exercise care here to not raise your shoulder/scapula when positioning your elbow or forearm against your waist. As this connection comes to feel more familiar, you can practice launching your right arm and fist forward, extending beyond that point where your elbow detaches from your waist. Try to feel the power expressed through your arm as stemming from your waist (Figure 5-67).

As before, whenever you wish to examine the quality of your connection, you can enlist the assistance of a partner to provide mild to moderate resistance against

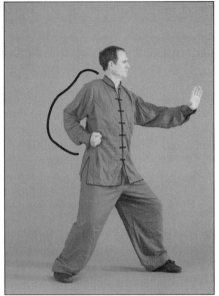

Figure 5-64a Avoid raising the shoulder . . .

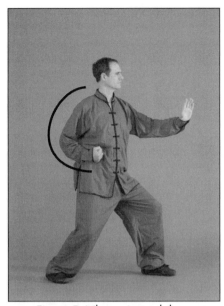

Figure 5-64b . . . instead, keep it relaxed.

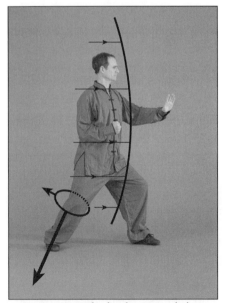

Figure 5-65 The back same-side leg propels the whole body forward.

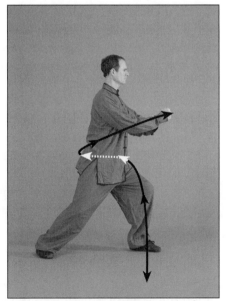

Figure 5-66 Arrows show how the forward opposite-side leg delivers power to the fist.

your fist (Figure 5-68). If no partner is available, you can lean with your fist against the nearest wall, tree, or whatever (Figure 5-69). Practice this skill until you have a replicable sense of moving force, starting from your leg, through your waist, and

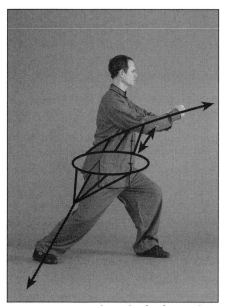

Figure 5-67 Launching the fist forward so the elbow separates from the waist.

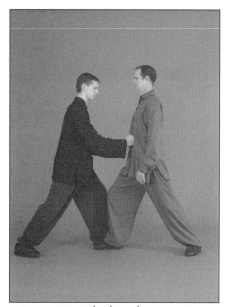

Figure 5-68 Checking the connection.

out through your arm and fist along an uninterrupted path. When you do this correctly your arm and waist should move as if they are a single unit.

Eventually, your skill will develop to a point that you will be able to move your arm just "offshore" from your waist, while maintaining this solid connection between your punching arm and your waist without actually connecting the two together (Figures 5-70a and b). I recommend, however, that you wait until after you have developed a thorough grasp of the earlier stages before experimenting with this "non-connected connection."

Getting back to my friend, after I had explained all this to her, she was able to practice it a few times, feeling the improvement in her connection immediately. She turned to me and asked if this

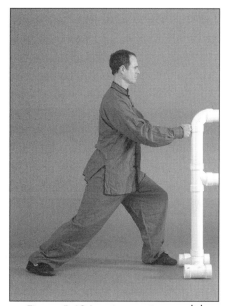

Figure 5-69 Leaning against a solid object when no partner is available.

specific guidance was included in my just released second book. "Actually, it's not," I confessed. "Well, it oughta be," she replied.

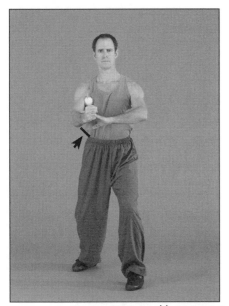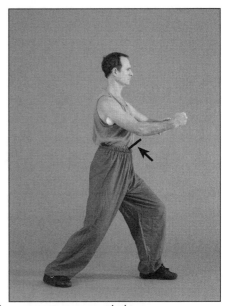

Figures 5-70a and b Maintaining the connection even with the arm positioned off the waist. Note tennis ball spacer in armpit.

Feeling Your Ward Off Connection

Among the most common flaws in technique that I observe in practitioners, even those who are more experienced, are lapses (or outright absences) in structural continuity. Structure is not merely an end point quality, such as might occur at the conclusion of a move. It is a dynamic to be observed throughout every move. I emphasize this point because students newer to Tai Chi are often held accountable for their structure in *only* that manner, as some quality they must display at the conclusion of this move or that. It is unfortunate then, but only natural, that the student's expression of his or her grasp of structure remains limited to the conclusion, or termination point, of individual techniques. From a practical point of view, being able to express a grasp of your connected structure only as a static quality, such as occurs at the endpoint of a move, is of little value other than as a bench mark along your path of learning.

A second important point is that your attention to good structure should permeate your form, and your practice overall, as a continuum. Your attention to the structural underpinning of any move or position must begin at its beginning and not merely occur at its terminus. In order for structure to be of practical value to you, it must be every bit as dynamic as the rest of your form. Your structure must constantly move, adapt, and readjust as your form and your body unfold from posture to posture.

In T'ai Chi there are certain essential, or cardinal, moves. The names of some of these moves denote specific positions while others suggest much more than any particular position. To illustrate these points, let's take a closer look at the move

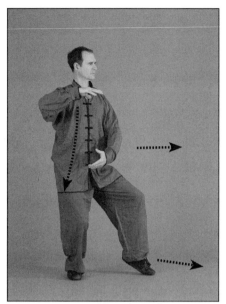

Figure 5-71a Holding the Ball in preparation for Ward Off.

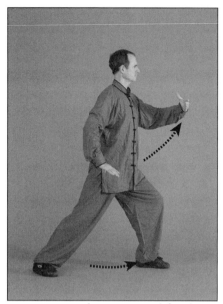

Figure 5-71b Moving into left-side Ward Off.

Ward Off. Ward Off, as a specific move, is usually practiced as one component of the sequence known as Grasp the Bird's Tail. Besides its occurrence as a clearly identifiable move, Ward Off is also a T'ai Chi essence. That is to say it represents a particular way in which energy, or force, is expressed in T'ai Chi Ch'uan. As an essence, Ward Off is not limited to the context of its namesake move, but occurs repeatedly throughout the T'ai Chi form in other moves. Because both the move Ward Off and the essence Ward Off play so prominently in T'ai Chi, it is instructive to highlight Ward Off, the move, in an effort to explain more clearly how you can accomplish structure both as a fluid dynamic in this particular move, and as an ongoing feature throughout your own T'ai Chi practice.

The Ward Off move usually unfolds and culminates into a posture (Figures 5-71a and b) on either the right or left side. As always, we are concerned with good structure, the quality of which in the finished position may be determined by engaging the assistance of a partner. A correctly structured position will hold steady under duress (Figure 5-72), while a poorly structured posture will fail to withstand even a moderate amount of stress (Figure 5-73).

Accomplishing a correct structure in your finished position is an important, albeit first, step in fully understanding your Ward Off connection. Accomplishing good structure at the end point of any move is also the easiest part of acquiring structure. Once you have a replicable sense of structure in this finished position, you will be ready to expand your grasp of the structural subtleties of Ward Off—backward through its earlier stages as well.

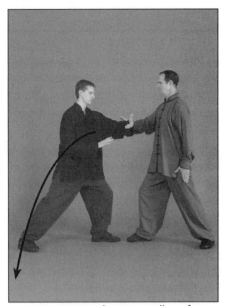

Figure 5-72 Good structure allows force to pass through to the earth . . . (note how Ward Off position has forward thumb extended upward to emphasize the arm's 'leading edge')

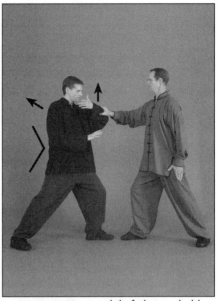

Figure 5-73 . . . while failure to hold under duress indicates poor structure.

To start, let's return to the very beginning of your Ward Off move, just at that point where you are preparing to step forward (Figure 5-74). It is here, even before you step, that you must take care to insure that your axillary (armpit) area is open and properly structured. Exactly at this stage of Ward Off, prior to actually stepping out, your primary focus and feeling of connection will center higher on your arm from your shoulder to your elbow (Figure 5-75). Figures 5-76a, b, and c illustrate how the positioning of your hand can also influence the structure of your arm. Uphold this quality of structure at your armpit as your stepping foot reaches out and touches, heel first, down to the floor

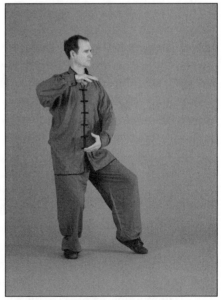

Figure 5-74 Preparing to step into Ward Off.

(Figure 5-77). As you begin to both shift your weight forward and lift and extend your leading arm, your arm's leading edge (refer to Figure 7-72) will be driven forward (Warding Off) by the full structure and momentum of the rest of your body.

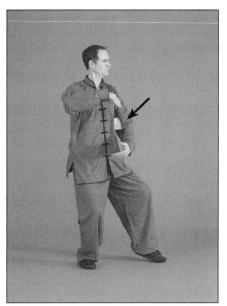

Figure 5-75 Structure is important during preparation (note spacer between arm and body).

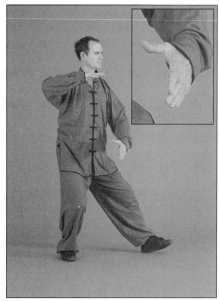

Figure 5-76a Incorrect: Palm turned facing too far in weakens arm structure (note thumb position in inset).

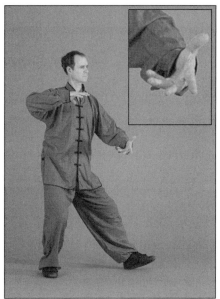

Figure 5-76b Incorrect: Palm turned facing too far out can also weaken arm structure (note thumb position in inset).

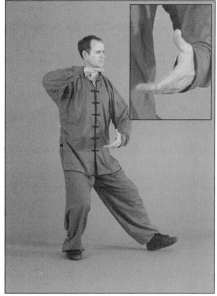

Figure 5-76c Correct: Palm facing slightly up enhances your arm and shoulder connection (note hand position in inset).

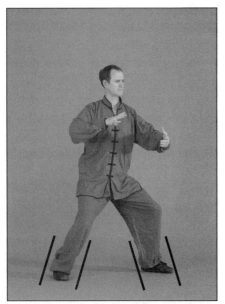

Figure 5-77 The heel and foot are planted down to prepare for Ward Off.

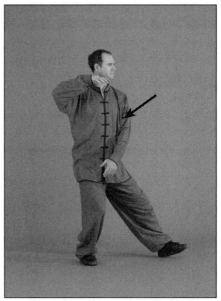

Figure 5-78 Arm too close so that the armpit is pinched shut.

A common error for beginners is to position the leading arm too close to the body so that the armpit is effectively pinched shut (Figure 5-78). Instead keep the armpit sufficiently open so that a tennis ball could fit comfortably in the gap (see Figure 5-79). Closing the armpit can pinch off the shoulder structure. If a partner (or opponent) pushes against your arm while your armpit is closed, you will have no means of redirecting his incoming force through your body and down to the earth. Instead, the force of his push will lodge in your shoulder and you will be an easy pushover (Figure 5-80). If, on the other hand, your armpit is open, as it should be, an incoming force can be deflected and redirected easily and harmlessly through your body and down to the earth (Figure 5-81).

Now, all you need do is maintain this same integrity of structure throughout your move. When your partner leans against you, as illustrated in Figure 5-81, the stability of your posture stems not from muscular resistance on your part, but from solid structural alignment. Your feeling of connection will be automatic, as if there were a support rod in place spanning the length of your upper arm (shoulder to elbow), and connecting directly to your tailbone. Your tailbone should feel, in turn, as if it is similarly braced down to your back foot (Figure 5-82). Once your back foot presses into the earth to drive your body forward, your imaginary brace will continue to feel as if it is adjusting automatically along your arm to provide support from your shoulder to your wrist (Figure 5-83). That's all there is to it. This concludes your Ward Off move.

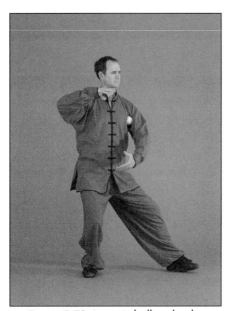

Figure 5-79 A tennis ball under the armpit helps set correct positioning.

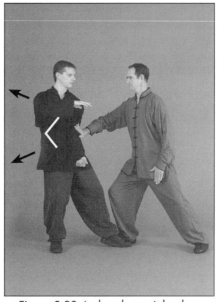

Figure 5-80 A closed armpit leads to instability . . .

By developing a clear comprehension of what connects to what, and why, you can streamline your grasp of this movement. Basing your movement on a clear understanding of your body's connections is much more efficient than random catch-as-catch-can, which is what usually happens when trying to acquire a skill through pure trial and error. Now you just need to practice until you feel the essence of your Ward Off connection as a continuum throughout your move. Keep in mind throughout that the greater part of whatever force you express through Ward Off stems not from your arm and shoulder, but initially from your legs and waist, and only subsequently through your arm and shoulder. Thus, the expression of Ward Off structure should be clear and unambiguous from the move's inception through to its conclusion.

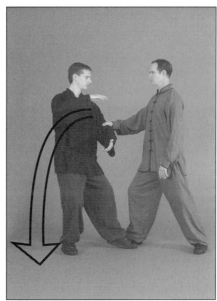

Figure 5-81 . . .while an open armpits allows for a transfer of force.

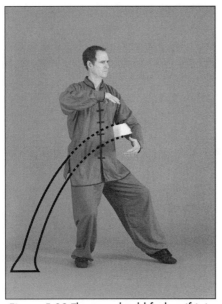

Figure 5-82 The arm should feel as if it is braced to the tailbone, and to the earth.

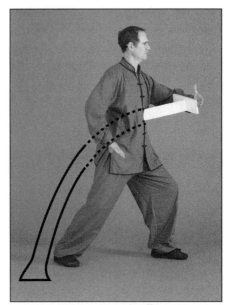

Figure 5-83 As Ward Off progresses forward, this 'brace' repositions.

How to Develop Spiraling Force—or the World is Our Screwdriver

I made a point earlier in this text of emphasizing that T'ai Chi's most defining quality is the manner in which it teaches us to negotiate the movement of force with the utmost of efficiency through our bodies. Usually, this calls to mind *earth force*, which travels from our feet upward, through our bodies, and outward to be issued via our upper body parts toward some target, real or imagined. Not all forces that pass through our bodies, though, come from the earth. Some forces, rather than coming from the earth and moving outward, may originate elsewhere, as when some other person issues force against you, and therefore force emanates from the outside in. The incoming force can be routed down through your body to the earth, or redirected past you into neutral space. Regardless of where a force comes from, in order for you to transfer it harmlessly through or past your body, you must be both sensitive to the force and have your body properly aligned. Otherwise, some or all of the force in question will put you in harm's way.

The nuances of dealing with "force in" versus "force out" require separate consideration. Depending on the nature and the intensity of an incoming force, your response may be as simple as "don't be there," or "get out of the way." The concept of "not being there," or emptiness, is a highly sought after skill in T'ai Chi. Despite the presumed higher skill level of being so empty that no one can hit you (a good strategy indeed for any incoming force!), it is actually more complicated, albeit less dangerous, to issue force outward than it is to receive it inwardly. This is because the proper issuance of force outward leaves less room for error, which may seem

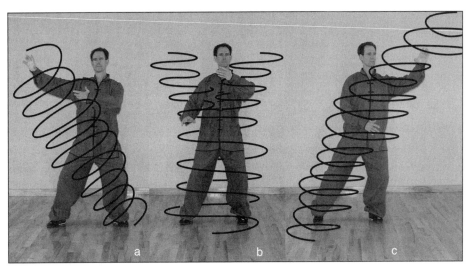

Figures 5-84a, b, and c These figures from my earlier book, Inside Tai Chi (Loupos 2002) were intended to depict the spiraling of earth force.

surprising at first. If you are on the receiving end of someone else's force, small errors or miscalculations can be compensated for, assuming the other person is not substantially more skilled than you. A lot can happen in a few fractions of a second. Your hands and arms are usually your first line of defense. But, if this first line of defense fails to detect or intercept an incoming force, you may still be able to neutralize that force at a next line of defense, at your shoulder, waist, etc. Or, you can absorb an incoming force and retreat, "hopping like a bird" as they say. However, when you initiate force, you alone are responsible for getting that force from the earth to its target, a goal that may be rendered even more challenging should your target be moving. But let's leave accuracy in tracking a moving target for another lecture.

The tricky part of issuing force out is to "spiral" it for mechanical efficiency. I wrote, briefly, about spiraling force in my first book (Loupos 2002, page 110) and depicted this concept with illustrations showing a series of concentric spirals moving from the earth upward and outward (Figures 5-84a, b, and c) Afterward, I had second thoughts about these illustrations because the graphics, if interpreted too literally, might seem to suggest that your force goes round and round your body prior to making its release. Not so. Actually, the process of spiraling force through your body is much subtler than those illustrations suggest. I would like to offer an alternate visualization to further clarify this important concept.

Developing spiraling power may be much easier if instead you can bring yourself to imagine your body as a giant screw. Imagining your body or any of its designated parts as a being threaded like a screw is actually a common enough concept that variations on this theme have been alluded to by many other teachers and writers. I employed a similar analogy several pages back when I discussed torquing the knee. Here, I would like you to imagine that your body is one big hardware screw. Think of yourself as one of those screws with a flat slotted head for a Phillips screwdriver. Now, think of your arms or your hands, or whatever body part you will issue your force through, as the pointed tip of the screw. Meanwhile, the head of the screw, where the screwdriver slots in to exert its turning and driving force, is at the sole of your foot. If the earth were a screwdriver, imagine it attaching to your foot, or feet, and torquing so as to drive force upward and outward through your body. It will be helpful here to keep in mind that the mechanics of a screw differ from those of a nail. A nail is made to work by being jolted forward by a sharp strike. A screw, on the other hand, is twisted spirally. It is the twisting of a screw (once its threads have bitten in) that actually causes it to pull itself forward into its target.

Indulge me for a moment here while I digress into a more detailed, and relevant, description of just how screws work. There are actually several different kinds of thread designs for screws, depending on their intended application. The two most familiar are common threads and machine threads. Common threads are more widely spaced apart (Figure 5-85), while machine screws have a much tighter thread weave (Figure 5-86). This means that the common screw, because its threads are wider apart, has fewer threads along its shaft. Therefore, fewer twists of the screwdriver are required to drive the screw fully into its target. A common screw's force is, thus, more aggressively impelling than that of a machine screw. However, your screwdriver must generate more torque in order to generate that impelling force. The tighter thread weave (meaning more threads) of the machine screw, requires relatively less force to advance the screw forward because each turn of the screwdriver results in less forward progress. Compared to the common screw, the force of a machine screw is less impelling, but because the machine screw has more and tighter threads it has the potential to attach more securely to its target.

How is this relevant to our topic? I find this distinction analogous to the variable manner in which we can use our bodies when employing spiraling force. Not all spiraling is the same. When issuing force through your body in a fashion comparable to a common screw your force has more *forward* drive. You opt for this kind of release when your intention is to impel force forward into your target and repel it back away from yourself in a straight line. This can most readily be seen in techniques such as Push or Press. A small twist of the screw, so to speak, creates a forward driving force.

In contrast, other techniques such as Rollback or Split entail a more deliberate engagement of your waist as a means of torquing your opponent off his center line. With techniques such as these, your intention may be to control your opponent, to manage or manhandle him, rather than simply repulse him. These techniques have a "tighter thread weave" and may require a bit more twisting of the screw, allowing you to exploit or borrow force from your opponent (which can then be

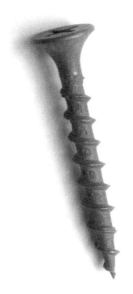
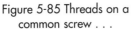
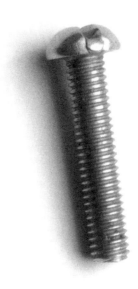

Figure 5-85 Threads on a
common screw . . .

Figure 5-86 . . . compared to threads of
a machine screw.

applied back against him). Consequently, whatever torquing force you generate can be issued against your opponent more with the idea of rerouting him than of repulsing him outright.

Now, getting back to the earth as your screwdriver, all you need in order to generate force for a powerful strike outward is a quarter turn or less, or for a rerouting force perhaps just a bit more of a twist. Most importantly, remember to draw your force from the earth, at your root, rather than muscling force through from your waist, back, or shoulders. In the next chapter we will examine in greater detail how to align your body so as to actually acquire this type of skill.

CHAPTER 6

Moving Force from Your Earth Root

Rootedness as a Foundation for Issuing Force

Learning how to root yourself is one of T'ai Chi's most essential skills. In fact, the quality of one's rootedness is often what separates more serious and accomplished T'ai Chi students from novices and casual practitioners. Attaining a feeling of rootedness or connectedness to the earth is an important milestone for students. I provided detailed guidance in my first book *Inside Tai Chi* (Loupos 2002) on how to acquire your root. Even so, having a sense of rootedness and then learning how to take full advantage of that rootedness for the purpose of issuing force outward from your body are two different matters. Rootedness itself is but a first step, so to speak. Before I proceed with guidance on an exercise designed to help you learn how to use your earth root connection specifically for issuing force outward, let me define my terms a bit.

For readers newer to T'ai Chi, the idea of "issuing force outward" may seem to have something of a martial connotation about it. Rest easy if you are not a fighter, as I don't mean to alienate those of you lacking a martial background, orientation, or ambition. The truth is that nearly everything you do with your body involves issuing force outward in some manner or another. Just getting yourself up and out of bed in the morning means you must issue force against the pull of the earth's gravity in order to stand up and not fall back down. Simple stepping, one foot after the other, involves your pushing force down against the earth, as do more complex tasks such as carrying your groceries in from the car, doing chores around the house, or riding your bicycle. In each case, it is necessary to push against the earth either directly as in walking or indirectly as in bicycling in order to move force, first through, and then from your body so as to propel yourself in any direction. Unless you are lying down, sitting immobile, or making use of isometric force or the like, the efficiency of whatever you are doing is ultimately dependent on how you connect to the earth. It would make sense then, given the global presence of this dynamic in your life, to get it right. As a T'ai Chi practitioner, you will want to transfer force through and from your body in a manner that is optimally efficient. Herein lies the great value of T'ai Chi, with its emphasis on form practice and auxiliary training methods. In this chapter, I will guide you in learning one of these auxiliary training methods as a means of moving force through your body with ease and efficiency.

Figuring out how to move force from the earth, through your body, upward and outward requires a specialized training that, by my way of thinking, is not adequately addressed by T'ai Chi form practice alone. This, of course, is why there have developed different kinds of auxiliary practices; various Push Hands patterns, standing meditations, Chi Kung practices, etc. Push Hands, as one example, enables you to engage with someone else's body and affords you a quality of feedback about your own body that solo practice simply cannot provide. Push Hands, depending on the pattern employed, both encourages the development of and reinforces a fairly broad range of T'ai Chi skills—skills that are both adjunct and complementary to form practice. During pushing practice, there may be a host of different skills, albeit related, that you are expected to be attentive to all at once if you are an experienced practitioner. As a newer learner, though, you must start slowly, acquiring each skill in turn. You can hardly expect, or be expected, to grasp the full range of skills required for pushing practice immediately.

Learning Push Hands is no different from any other undertaking that involves hands-on learning. In order for your knowledge and understanding of the subject to be based on a solid foundation, you must first acquire experience through practice. Prior to gaining that experience, you may find yourself inclined to randomly, or instinctively, focus your attention on this T'ai Chi quality or that, or even on several qualities at once. With continued practice and guidance from your teacher you will begin to develop an appreciation for the learning hierarchy in the skills involved. For example, a tendency to focus your attention inordinately on aligning your body for the issuance of force may need to yield its position to the development of softness, or "listening" (*ting jin*), or moving from your *dantien*, or adhering to your partner, etc. As a rule, the exact order of the skills involved in the T'ai Chi learning hierarchy is inexact. Students vary in their abilities and T'ai Chi teachers vary in how they prioritize the many aspects of their art.

Thus, the T'ai Chi learning hierarchy is flexible and fluid. The best way to approach this particular learning depends on a number of factors perhaps best left to your teacher to interpret. I will say, though, that as ambitious as you may be to grasp all these various skills and get them properly coordinated, it is best to proceed slowly and undertake them one skill at a time. Oftentimes it is easier to acquire a particular skill if you are able to confine the fuller focus of your attention to just that one skill. Breaking down your practice in a way that allows you to focus on one skill at a time can be an effective way to assemble, over time, all the building blocks of good T'ai Chi. Practicing to develop individual building blocks can strengthen your foundation and also afford you a clearer and more complete understanding of what you are doing and why. In the long run, an approach such as this is what helps you to assume full ownership of your T'ai Chi.

One particular training method that I rely on in class helps students to feel their bodies align in just the right way, so they can actually feel an efficient transfer of force from the earth upward and outward. On the one hand, prearranged Push Hands generally involves prescribed classical patterns. On the other hand, Push Hands can be whatever partner practice you engage in that teaches you pushing hand skills. I don't regard the exercise that follows as a Push Hands pattern, not in the classical sense, because its emphasis is almost exclusively geared toward transferring force efficiently. At least in its early stages, this exercise entails relatively less attention to *Ting Jin* or to softness, qualities which are generally characteristic of Push Hands practice. Regardless, this method offers a ready means for students of all levels to feel what it is like to guide force through their bodies in the easiest and most efficient manner.

The directions that follow for this exercise may seem complicated at first. My instructions will guide you in shifting your body into different positions whilst you (eventually) engage the cooperation of a partner who is not doing exactly the same thing at the same time as you are. Because of this, all the usual challenges commensurate with trying to convey the intricacies of a moving pattern in a book using still photos will apply. Nevertheless, I will try to be as clear and succinct as possible so that you can try your hand at this exercise. Take it slow, one step at a time, and the benefits of this practice will make it well worth the effort entailed in learning it.

Your ideal partner for learning this exercise will be someone who is about your own height and weight. Size or height discrepancies between partners can be beneficially challenging once your skill level is more advanced. At the beginning, however, it is best to work with someone about your own size.

Getting Started: Part 1

I will describe each partner's role individually, and in detail, prior to describing the roles of both partners together. The terms *clockwise* and *counter clockwise* have the potential to be misleading as they are perspective dependent. For the purpose of clarity, and unless noted otherwise, my descriptions will stem from the perspective of being positioned behind the partner designated as the *aggressor*. In your imagination, you will be following the aggressor as if from behind, thus sparing yourself any need to reverse or otherwise reconfigure in your mind the instructions given.

Partner A (that's you), in what will initially be the aggressor role, begins by standing as shown in Figures 6-1a and b, positioned in a left foot forward leaning stance, with both your arms hanging freely. Be careful here to employ a slightly modified version of your usual forward leaning stance, so that the width of your stance is narrower than usual (Figure 6-2). Your feet should remain nearly aligned with each other throughout this exercise. The basic idea of this drill will be for you

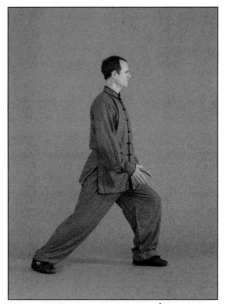

Figure 6-1a Partner A in ready position, viewed from the open side . . .

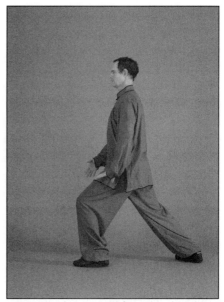

Figure 6-1b . . . .and from the closed, or back, side.

to move your right arm in a full circle, arcing it clockwise from its starting position at six o'clock past seven o'clock, eight o'clock, and so on, all the way back around to six o'clock (Figures 6-3a, b, c, and d). Note how the palm is positioned facing inward, toward your body, during the first half of the arc, and away from your body during the second phase (see insets). It is quite important that you establish and maintain a feeling of full extension from your shoulder all the way out to your fingertips throughout this pattern. Pay special attention to this feeling of extension from eleven o'clock through one o'clock. Also, any stiffness in your shoulder may cause it to scrunch up and restrict the full extension of your arm; so be careful as your arm arcs up

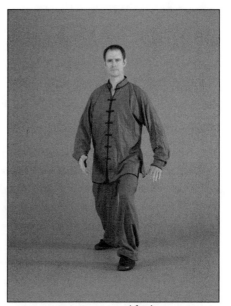

Figure 6-2 Use a modified, narrower than usual leaning stance.

overhead that your shoulder stays relaxed and settled down (Figures 6-4a and b). Part 1 for your side concludes as your right arm arcs all the way over and around to six o'clock.

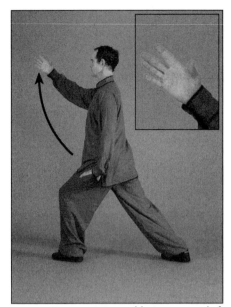
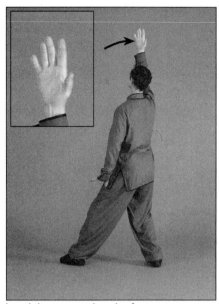

Figures 6-3a and b Arm extends forward and then up, with palm facing in.

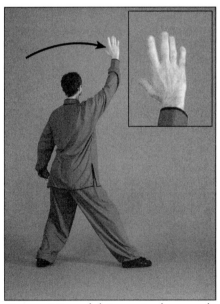
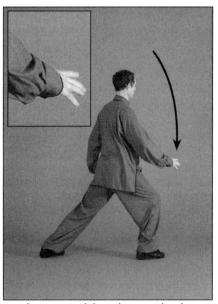

Figures 6-3c and d Arm extends upward and out (palm out) and then down (palm down).

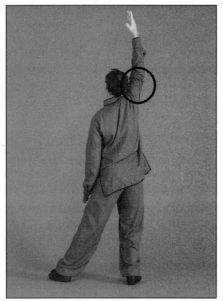

Figure 6-4a Incorrect: shoulder is lifted.

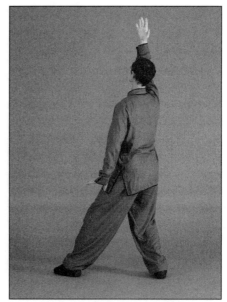

Figure 6-4b Correct: shoulder remains relaxed.

Part 2, will entail partner A (still you) reversing direction and moving your same (right) arm counter-clockwise from six o'clock, past five o'clock, and so on, extending all the way up, over, and back to your starting position at six o'clock. However, before we tackle part 2, let's back up for just a moment to the beginning of part 1. To avoid the confusion that would have ensued had I given you too many details to focus on at one time, I deliberately omitted the directions for the accompanying footwork. Now that you have the pattern for your arm movements, we need to add in that footwork prior to reversing our pattern.

Prepare, once again, to commence the movements as outlined above from your ready position. This time, push

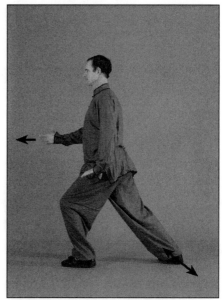

Figure 6-5 Push into the right foot to extend the right arm forward.

down into your back (right) foot to create an impetus for extending your right arm forward along its upward, clockwise arc (Figure 6-5). As your arm extends up toward eleven o'clock, begin to push less with your back foot and more with your

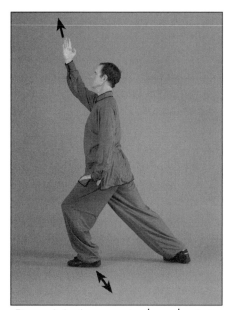

Figure 6-6a As arm extends up, begin to sink back.

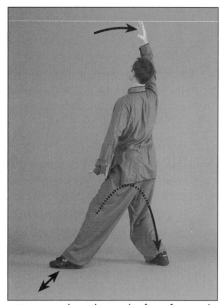

Figure 6-6b Push into the front foot and sink fully into the tail bone and back leg.

front (left) foot (Figure 6-6a). As you feel yourself pushing into your forward foot begin to sink your weight back and down into your tailbone. The timing of this is such that as the bulk of your weight shifts from your front foot to your back foot, your right arm should simultaneously extend from eleven o'clock around to one o'clock (Figure 6-6b).

Just as your extending hand passes twelve o'clock, begin to shift whatever weight you have remaining on your front foot from your front toes back onto your same side (left) heel. With the front part of your front foot unweighted, pivot your left foot on its heel clockwise around to the right (Figure 6-7a and b). Notice how the turning of your left foot turns your left leg, which should then turn your waist, which then turns your body, all the way 180 degrees around to the right. At the same time that you are turning your leg and body, you should also rotate your right arm, so that its palm is facing outward and away from your body. Your right palm should complete this rotation outward as it arcs between one o'clock and two o'clock (Figure 6-8). Just as your palm turns outward so must your right foot now rotate fully forward, so that you are now in a right foot forward leaning stance. Continue extending your right arm along its arc until it reaches six o'clock. You should now be positioned in a near mirror image of your starting position (Figures 6-9a and b).

Obviously, there are a great many details to attend up to this point. Before proceeding, I recommend that you pause and linger here and practice until you feel competent in your ability to follow along with the instructions. This is a complex

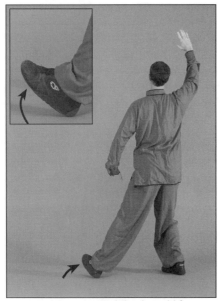

Figure 6-7a Sink back and lift
the toes . . .

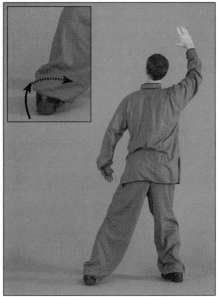

Figure 6-7b . . . and turn the
foot inward.

movement; so take it slow and practice one detail at a time until you are able to synchronize all the details.

The Return Trip: Part 2

Now we will begin to reverse the pattern with part 2. Sorry to say, the return trip is not quite as simple as doing everything you just did in part 1 in mirror image. Previously, the arm that you moved corresponded at first to your back foot: right arm together with right foot. Now, as you begin part 2 using that same right arm, your starting position has your opposite (left) foot to the rear instead of your right foot (Figure 6-10). This will require some modifications as you prepare to arc your leading arm and rotate your body counter-clockwise, back around to its original starting position.

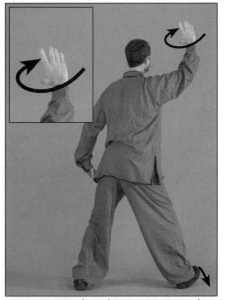

Figure 6-8 Right palm rotates outward at
between 1 o'clock and 2 o'clock.

Begin by pressing your left (back) foot down against the earth to provide a forward impetus that will extend your right arm forward and up (Figure 6-11). Try to

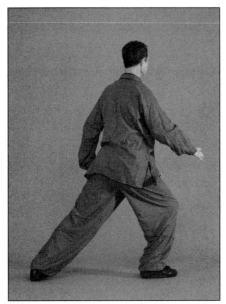

Figure 6-9a Arm arc and stance transition completed, back view . . .

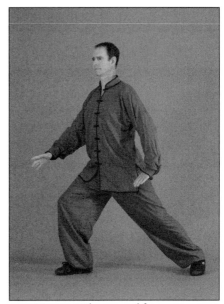

Figure 6-9b . . . and front view.

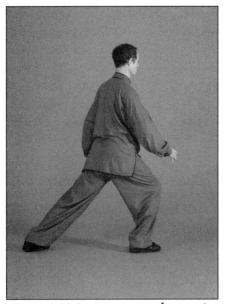

Figure 6-10 Starting position for part 2,
with left foot to the rear.

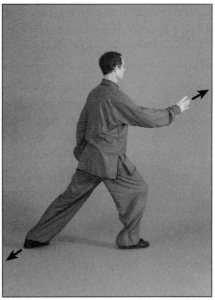

Figure 6-11 Pressing back into the left
foot and extending the right arm forward.

sustain the feeling of this earthbound connection through your foot as your right
arm with its palm facing to front extends as far as possible away from that foot. At
that point, when your right arm reaches a 180-degree extension away from your

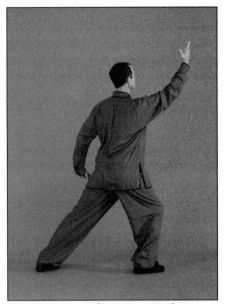

Figure 6-12 Right arm is 180 degrees away from back leg, between one and two o'clock.

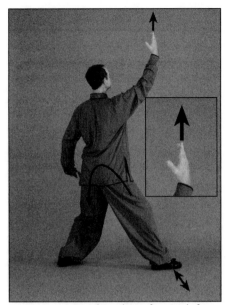

Figure 6-13 Right palm is forward, fingers extending (see inset).

back leg, your arm should be aiming at between one o'clock and two o'clock (Figure 6-12). From this point, your emphasis will begin to shift from pushing forward with your back leg to pushing upward and backward off your front leg, while simultaneously sinking back into your tailbone and back leg. All the while, as your right arm arcs up overhead, the fingertips of your right hand should continue to extend away from your body (Figure 6-13).

As your right arm extends upward toward twelve o'clock, you should begin to shift the bulk of the weight on your front foot from its toes back onto its heel. Once the front part of your foot is unweighted you can peel your toes up and begin to turn your right foot inward, counter clockwise around to the left. This, in turn, will spiral your right leg around, and then your waist, and along with your waist the rest of your body. As your right foot turns and plants firmly down, you should turn your left foot straight forward to the left, and sink the bulk of your weight into your now forward (left) leg. Simultaneously, as you shift your feet, legs, and body 180 degrees around to the left, your right arm will rotate its palm under and inward as if you were preparing to chop down with the knife edge of that hand. Maintain the feeling of extending your fingers outward away from your body (Figures 6-14a, b, c, and d) and continue extending until your arm reaches six o'clock. Avoid lifting your shoulder throughout (Figure 6-14e). Congratulations! This completes part 2.

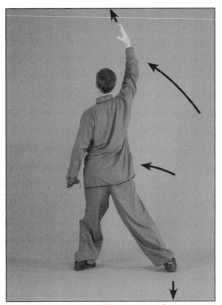
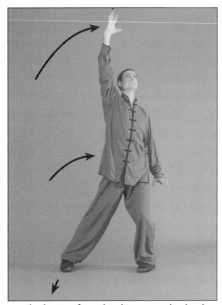

Figures 6-14a and b Moving the arm in a counter-clockwise (from back) arc as the body turns left (back and front views). Palm starts to rotate inward at twelve o'clock . . .

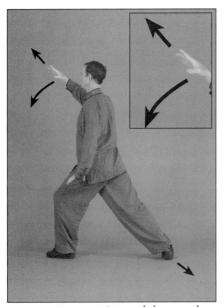
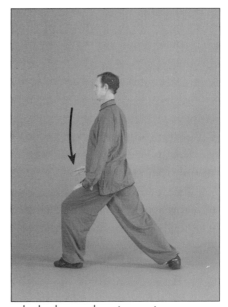

Figures 6-14c and d . . . and turns in as the body completes its rotation. Inset shows position of palm as the body turns.

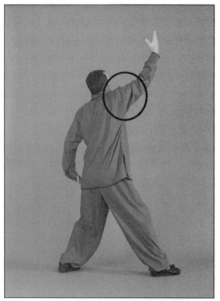

Figure 6-14e Be careful throughout to not lift the shoulder as shown.

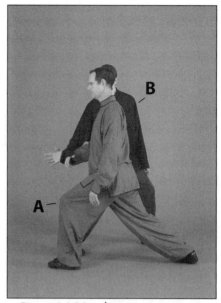

Figure 6-15 Ready to start. Partner A from the back, partner B opposite.

Again, I have saddled you with some fairly complex instructions. And, again, I recommend that you pause here. Take your time and practice, detail by detail, everything we have covered up until this point before you continue. After a few rounds of practice, this sequence will feel much less complicated.

Putting It All Together

Now that you have learned parts 1 and 2, it is time to put this together with your training partner. From here on it is as simple as coordinating your side of what you have just learned with your partner's side. You, as the aggressor, will start right back at the very beginning with your right wrist positioned inside (beneath) your partner's right wrist. For ease of reference, we will designate your partner B as the resister (see Figure 6-15).

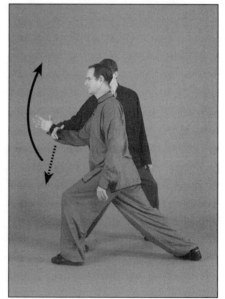

Figure 6-16 The partner offers a measured resistance. The solid arrow shows A's path of travel. The broken line indicates B's resistance.

As the aggressor, you need only follow exactly the directions previously outlined for

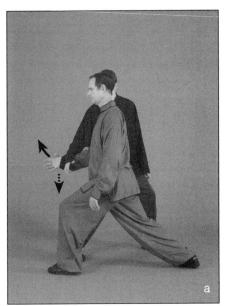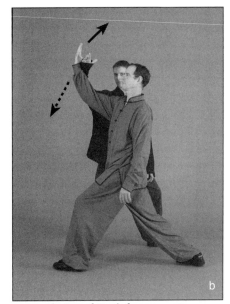

Figures 6-17a and b. From starting position to conclusion of Earth force exercise.

part 1. While you are enacting part 1 your partner will be assuming the more passive role by providing a measured resistance against your efforts to arc your arm up
and over (see Figure 6-16).

How much resistance your partner applies against your efforts is something the
both of you will need to agree on beforehand, lest you end up in a wrestling match,
or worse. I recommend that you start with negligible resistance and gradually work
up to just enough resistance to provide some challenge, but not a struggle. A light
to moderate resistance by partner B will encourage you, as the aggressor, to stay
focused in the moment and to not falter in the structural connections underlying
your movement. Remember, this is an exercise designed to promote good structure
as a means of facilitating the efficient transfer of earth force through your body. It
is not meant to be a contest of strength.

Once you and your partner have completed part 1, you will notice that you are
both in an (almost) exact mirror image of your original starting position. However,
your right wrist is now situated atop your partner's wrist, rather than underneath as it
was at the beginning of your drill. No matter. (In point of fact, you and your partner
have now reversed roles.) Your partner will assume the role of the aggressor. He will
become partner A, and you, now as partner B, will provide the resistance. In this manner, the two of you can go back and forth as many times as you like. Refer to the photos (Figures 6-17a, b, c, d, and e) for a full round, from one side to the other and back.

After you have had ample practice with one side (both of you using your right
arm), you can both switch to your other arms and repeat the pattern. Even as you

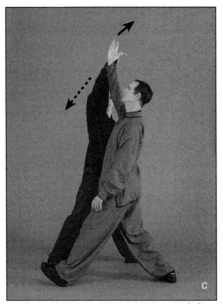
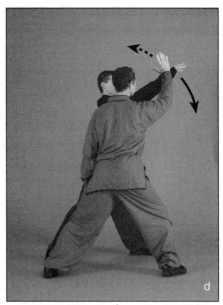

Figures 6-17c and d. Earth force exercise (continued).

and your partner both alternate arms, your footwork and legwork will remain uniform throughout.

Possible Problems

There are two basic concerns, which may be problematic for whoever is the aggressing partner A. The first of these includes problems that the aggressor may cause to himself due to flawed technique (more on this shortly). The second concern involves ploys on his resisting partner B's part that may serve to foil the aggressor's technique. While each partner is taking his turn as the aggressor A and preparing to move force from the earth in opposition to his partner B's resistance, the resisting partner has the reciprocal opportunity to neutralize and undermine

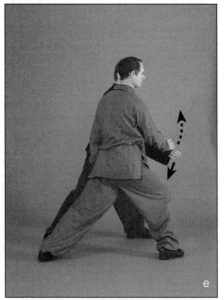

Figure 6-17e. Earth force exercise (continued).

the aggressor's force, in effect to render partner A ineffectual. Happily, every problem has a solution, and it is the process, and challenge, of figuring out these solutions according to the T'ai Chi principles of softness and yielding, versus strength and rigidity, that will improve your sensitivity and bring about improvement in your overall level of skill.

The role of the more passive resisting partner B is really quite easy. Foiling the aggressor's technique, as it is described in the earlier section, simply involves *splitting* A's structure. Done correctly, this will require very little effort on your part. Splitting is actually a more refined (and therefore preferable) skill compared to using muscular force to overpower the aggressor's efforts. Remember, in T'ai Chi we always try to employ the least amount of force necessary to accomplish a task. Splitting, at least in the context of this exercise, requires that the "splitter" stay relaxed rather than expend any appreciable amount of effort. The secret to splitting the aggressor's force with such relative ease lies, first, in reading his body structure, and then simply either leaning into any weak or vulnerable hollow areas or borrowing force from protruding areas. Thus, the task and the challenge for the aggressor A is to remain connected throughout and not give the resisting partner B any weakness or vulnerabilities to exploit. This is easier said than done. Once you reach the stage where these concerns have presented themselves and been satisfactorily resolved, your practice will be more akin to an actual Push Hands pattern.

Remember, as the aggressor your main goal will be to keep your body, and especially your arm, connected throughout, without any weak links in your structural continuum. In order to accomplish this, you must stay beneath your resisting partner's force. Staying "below his radar" is a task you must accomplish even when your hand is positioned atop your partner's hand. Even while your hand may be, technically, atop that of your partner, you can still keep your energetic center below his energetic center and maintain a "lifting and leading" impetus with your arcing arm. In this manner you can maintain a structural advantage. I will provide two examples of the problems just described, but resolving all these issues as they arise is something you will need to experiment with in collaboration with your partner.

The first potential problem area occurs right at the beginning of the exercise, just as you prepare to engage your leading arm. At this point the resisting partner may thwart your efforts simply by relaxing (sinking) his weight through his arm down against your arm (see Figure 6-18). If you take the bait, so to speak, and struggle back against his lean, you will almost surely lift your shoulder in the process and so render yourself "split" (Figure 6-19). Being "split" means that a force of yours that you intend to go in one direction has ruptured into two or more directions.

Instead of struggling back, you as the aggressor must relax and settle under the resister's hand by extending first down and out rather than forward and up (Figures 6-20a and b). This, in effect, *splits* the resister's attempt to *split* you. Again, the emphasis here is on refinement and finesse rather than brute force.

Try to feel your body expanding and extending in order to avoid flaws in your structure that your partner might try to exploit. The feeling of expanding and

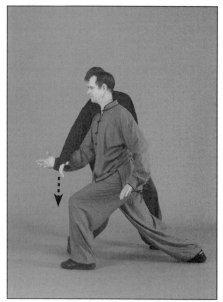

Figure 6-18 The resister (opposite) merely leans against the aggressor's hand.

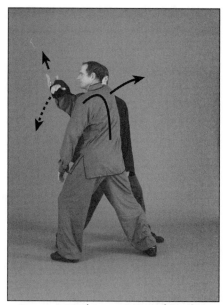

Figure 6-19 This aggressor's force has been split in two directions.

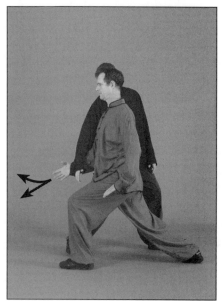

Figure 6-20a Extending down and out to stay under a partner's resistance. . .

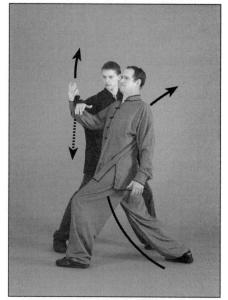

Figure 6-20b . . .instead of reaching forward and up.

extending starts with your fingers, by expanding your finger joints, and ranges all the way back through your body to your earth connection at your feet. Even if you are shorter of limb than your partner, it is still possible for you to extend in a way that prevents his splitting your force, providing you maintain proper structure.

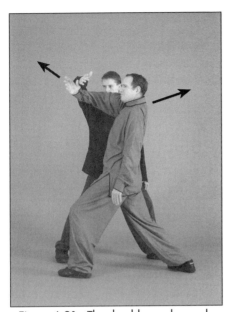

Figure 6-21a The shoulder and scapula lifting up incorrectly . . .

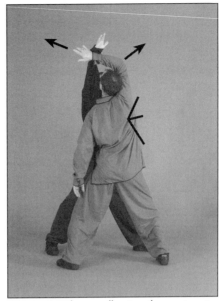

Figure 6-21b . . . allowing the partner to split the force.

The second potential problem area occurs in the overhead portion of your move, just as your and your partner's arms pass between eleven o'clock and one o'clock. At this critical juncture, you are extending your arm up and over whilst you reposition your stance and turn your body—all at the same time. There are two special challenges here. First, you must open your shoulder without lifting it as you continue to extend your arm upward. Even as your fingers extend skyward, you must relax your same side scapula down in order to maintain its connection to your tailbone and feet. If you make the mistake of raising your shoulder your partner will surely sense the resultant weakness and neutralize your efforts by splitting your shoulder force (Figures 6-

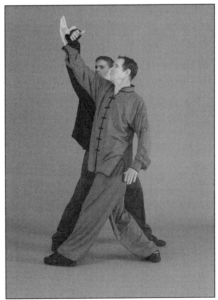

Figure 6-21c The scapula staying properly connected.

21a, b and c). Second, the timing of all these transitions (leg, waist, body, and arm) must be perfectly synchronized, lest your partner split you at any one of these juncture points (Figures 6-22a and b, 6-23a and b, 6-24a and b, 6-25a and b).

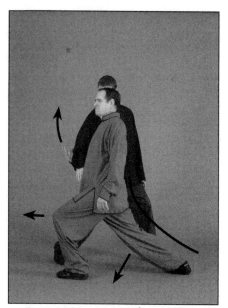

Figure 6-22a Incorrect leg structure.

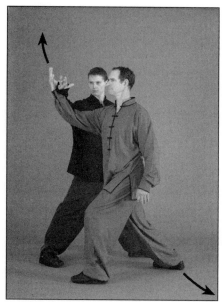

Figure 6-22b Correct leg structure.

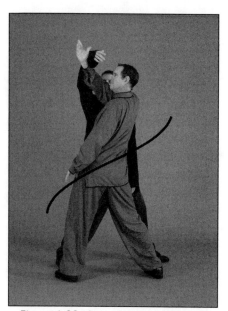

Figure 6-23a Incorrect waist structure.

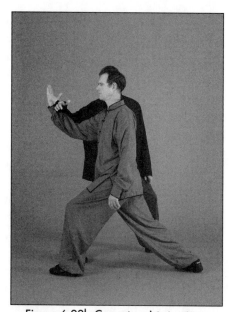

Figure 6-23b Correct waist structure.

These problems areas aside, success at this exercise is largely a matter of refining your skill and sensitivity through practice. Simply put, as you try to stay properly connected, your partner will try to split your force wherever your technique may be flawed. This is his or her way of helping you learn and improve your skill.

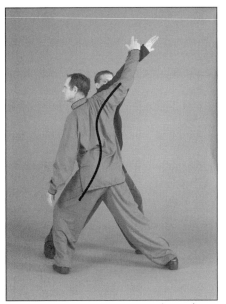

Figure 6-24a Incorrect torso/scapular structure.

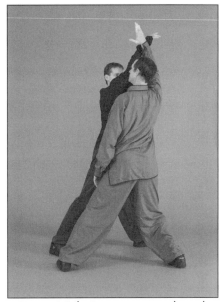

Figure 6-24b Correct structure through torso and scapula.

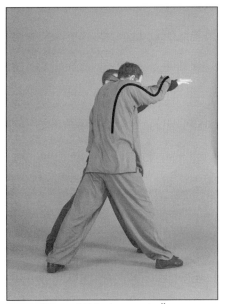

Figure 6-25a Incorrect elbow and wrist structure

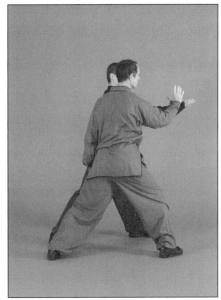

Figure 6-25b Correct arm structure.

Then you reverse roles, and it becomes your turn to split. In this way, each of you can improve your sense of structure while issuing force from the earth, as well as your sensitivity to structural nuances and vulnerabilities in an opponent who may be attempting to use force against you.

Points to Remember:

- Acquiring rootedness is but a first step in learning how to issue force.
- Form practice alone is inadequate for learning issue force.
- Confine your attention to learning one skill at a time.
- Start with a partner about your own size.
- When aggressing, maintain a feeling of extension throughout your move.
- When resisting, relax throughout your move.
- Agree, beforehand, with your partner how much resistance/force to apply.
- The process of arriving at a solution is, itself, a solution of sorts.
- Try to stay "beneath" your partner and lead him without fighting back for best advantage.
- Develop sensitivity to structural nuances.

CHAPTER *7*

The Role of Momentum in T'ai Chi

I could have chosen to write about the role of momentum in the context of T'ai Chi from any one of several possible angles. I might have opted for momentum as it occurs in Push Hands, or the momentum of your progress at your studies, or how T'ai Chi fits into the momentum of your life. Here, I have chosen to explore the more obvious manifestation of momentum as a dynamic in how you move your body during form practice.

Momentum is Unavoidable

Momentum is an unavoidable fact of life. Anytime you shift your body in one direction or another, there is a certain momentum that accompanies your movement. This is in accordance with Newton's first law of motion: *Every object in a state of uniform motion tends to remain in that state of motion unless an external force is applied to it.* However, not all momentum is the same. In the context of T'ai Chi practice, I stipulate a distinction between momentum that is automatic and unconscious, as compared to momentum that has a basis in mindfulness and intent. It is, therefore, how we use our momentum that determines it propriety. Even though all movement carries with it a certain momentum, in T'ai Chi we seek to minimize our reliance on momentum as a dictating factor in how our technique unfolds. Rather, we T'ai Chi'ers should prefer that any momentum be incidental to our movement and only in consequence to mindful attention and intention.

Mind you, there is nothing inherently wrong with momentum. But in T'ai Chi you do not want your body's movements to be unduly influenced by inertia. It would not be in keeping with the principles of T'ai Chi if you were to allow any force other than that occasioned by your own conscious and deliberate intention to dictate how your body performs. To do so would be a glaring example of having your body "out of the moment." Momentum should never be inadvertent.

In T'ai Chi, as elsewhere in life, any movement you initiate will produce a certain momentum. During T'ai Chi practice, you want to use that momentum only to augment the movement that initiated it, not to supersede it. Whatever momentum you generate should be caused *by* your movement, and not the other way around. It is perfectly okay for momentum to drive the delivery of your technique, but momentum ought not to take on a life of its own. Why? Because momentum implies commitment to a course of action. And the kind of commitment that stems from momentum, as per Newton's first law, can be difficult to revoke. Momentum that has assumed a life of its own generally precludes adaptation and spontaneity, which are qualities that all T'ai Chi students aspire to. Momentum does have a place in T'ai Chi, but only by design.

Unfortunately, renouncing momentum is a task more easily said than accomplished. This is a fact that, coincidentally, serves as a premise for the famous saying in the *Taijiquan Classics*, that "An attack of one thousand catties can be deflected by a force of four taels."* The one thousand pound force being referred to is nothing more than some hapless attacker's momentum. The reason such a force can be so predictably deflected has as much to do with the attacker's feckless momentum as it does with the neutralizing skill of the T'ai Chi defender. Note, the operative word in the saying, as it has often been interpreted, is "*can* be deflected," not "*will* be deflected." This adage might read very differently if another T'ai Chi master was behind the momentum and his momentum was appropriate to the technique. The more inappropriate momentum there is behind an assault as it hurtles toward you, the less force (perhaps even just four taels) will be required to deflect it aside. This classic saying is usually interpreted as intended to teach and inspire from the perspective of the defender, the guy with four taels. Naturally, we would all like to be good enough to rely on just four taels. But you also want to take care to not be like that also-ran attacker whose fate seems so prophetically sealed in adage by his unbridled momentum.

Momentum in Lieu of . . .

Like so many other impairments to T'ai Chi, momentum is usually a compensatory dynamic. Momentum is often employed, albeit unconsciously, as a substitute for good technique and, as well, in compensation for its absence. If your body lacks a strong foundation in muscle and tendon support, or if your joints are not open and flexible to a point that they allow for pinpoint precision and control, momentum may be what you inadvertently rely on where good technique is wanting.

As with most problems, the first step in realizing a solution is to recognize what the problem is and where exactly it occurs. We have identified this problem. Now to locate it. Should you have occasion to scrutinize someone else's T'ai Chi form for flaws, you will find that you need to develop a discerning eye (or, in the case of your own form, a refined sensitivity), in order to distinguish between appropriate and inappropriate momentum (more on this shortly). And, as you might expect, good posture and rooting skills will play their usual crucial roles in determining whether or not you will be able to place a check on momentum in your own prac-

---

*1 catty, or jin, equals .5 kilogram, or 1.1 pounds. At the time the Classics were written, 16 taels, or liang, equaled approximately 1 ounce, equaled 1 catty. Currently, due to an updated system of weights and measures in China, 10 taels are regarded as equaling 1 catty.

tice. Bearing this in mind, I believe that remedying the underlying causes of momentum is a task that may be best dealt with only after you have acquired a solid grasp of other skills, i.e., rooting and properly aligned posture, requisite to high quality T'ai Chi. Accordingly, those readers who stand to gain the greatest benefit from the advice that follows are those who are already well experienced at their T'ai Chi practice.

Though we continually strive to eliminate flaws in our practice, the momentum that occurs inadvertently during form practice, at least as far as beginners are concerned, is probably not T'ai Chi's worst evil, my earlier condemnation of momentum notwithstanding. Because inappropriate momentum is not so much a problem itself as it is an expression of other weaknesses or flaws, it may just be that momentum is a minor fault that you will have to live with until you develop the skills necessary to obviate its role in your practice. In fact, recognition of momentum can actually be a blessing to the extent that it points the way to its deeper and more fundamental causations. More often than not, less experienced students lack the basic awareness of self that is requisite to sensing misalignments or imbalances in their bodies. Because they lack this sensitivity, their subtler underlying problems can elude detection over years or even decades of practice. Learning how to recognize momentum, however, can be much easier than recognizing more deeply seated imbalances. Even less experienced students can easily learn to recognize momentum where it occurs, which can then lead them to ferret about for underlying causes. Subsequently, as they learn to eliminate those causes, they will, by default, eliminate their momentum. This then is but one more example of "investing in loss." Even though it may be premature, especially if you are a novice at T'ai Chi, to focus inordinately on eliminating momentum from your own practice, there is no harm in discussing corrective measures, regardless of where you are in the scheme of your training.

Factors other than inexperience can also contribute to inadvertent momentum. Just how obvious momentum might present in any given practitioner can depend on age and also on athletic talent (or, more correctly, somatic intelligence). The proprioceptive function in youthful practitioners or in students who are athletically gifted may afford them a more reliable feedback about where their bodies are at all times. Consequently, students who still have the proprioception of youth or who are gifted with a high degree of somatic intelligence may be better able to compensate for small lapses in balance (that is, "get away" with momentum) as allowances can, apparently, be made for minor indiscretions caused by momentum. However, the downside is that this can, in a sense, "enable" these practitioners, making them less prone to recognize momentum for the problem that it is in the first place, or even at all. The irony here is that not only is momentum compensatory in nature, but it is not always easily recognizable as a problem because naturally gifted practitioners can compensate for it by adapting to the problem. I don't

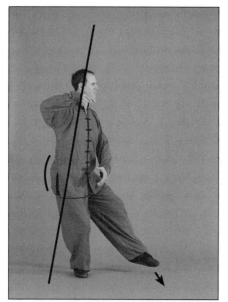 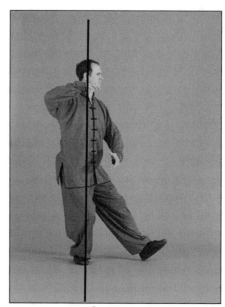

Figure 7-1a Incorrect: Falling out
into Ward Off.

Figure 7-1b Correct: Stepping
into Ward Off.

mean to suggest here that momentum is never a problem for younger or naturally gifted practitioners, only that appearances can mislead to suggest that momentum is an easily managed problem of minor consequence.

With the natural decline in proprioception that occurs with the aging process, momentum becomes more of a concern as we grow older. Older folks, for whom proprioceptive feedback may be less reliable, are less able to compensate for inertial errors. Of course, if you don't correct momentum as a younger practitioner, you run the risk that it will be thoroughly ingrained as an unproductive practice pattern by the time you are older.

To whatever extent it is possible to do so with still photos, the following illustrations (Figures 7-1a through 7-5a) compare individuals caught in momentum-based transitions with those who are transitioning correctly, moving from their roots and through their centers. You can use these comparisons as a guide to help you discern where your own techniques may be remiss.

Rid Your Form of Momentum

Enough already with theory! Assuming you are ready, how are you now going to reign in your momentum? Probably the easiest and most effective way to test for the occurrence of inappropriate momentum in your form is to experiment with the pacing of your moves. If you have settled into any sort of complacent groove with your practice, as most students tend to do, there is a good chance that your movements are (unbeknownst to you) premised at least somewhat on momentum. Try

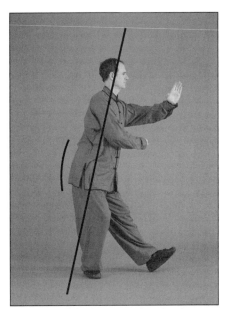

Figure 7-2a Incorrect: Leaning into
Fist Under Elbow.

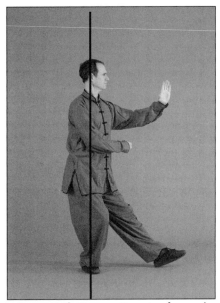

Figure 7-2b Correct: Stepping forward
with balance.

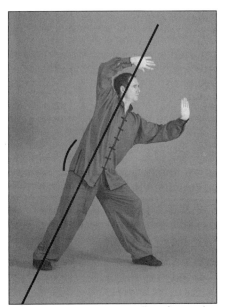

Figure 7-3a Incorrect: Falling forward
into Fan Through Back.

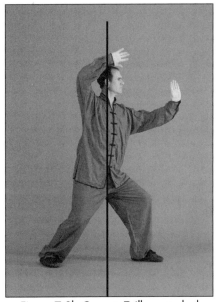

Figure 7-3b Correct: Tailbone tucked
under allows for a balanced advance.

slowing your form down a couple of notches and pay close attention to places where
you experience resistance or difficulty due to practicing more slowly. If each of the
movements you perform is properly founded in good structure and technique then

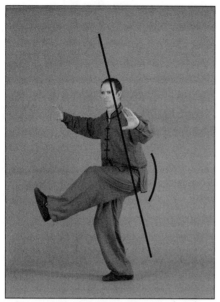

Figure 7-4a Incorrect: Parry and Kick.

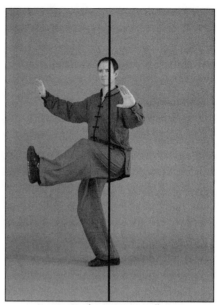

Figure 7-4b Correct: Tailbone tilted under.

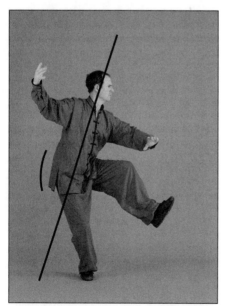

Figure 7-5a Incorrect: Falling forward to recover from Separate and Kick.

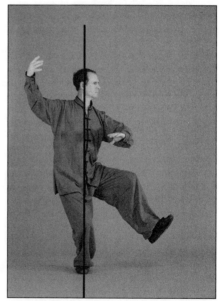

Figure 7-5b Correct: Advancing while maintaining a center line

you should have little difficulty executing your moves correctly, regardless of your speed. But, if you find that some movements are more challenging to perform well at your slower pace, then it is likely that you have discovered pockets of momentum where there should be none. Any such places beg closer scrutiny as they can point you to the underlying causes so that you can question and adjust your technique as necessary.

A variant on the approach just described is for you to stop—just freeze your movement—at random points throughout your form. Obviously, there are limits to this approach. Stopping in your tracks would not be practical, or advisable, during movements such as Turn (Spin) Around and Kick or as you are winding up for your Double Lotus Kick, as these moves are premised on momentum that is appropriate to the technique. This sort of technique aside, most other techniques and transitions do lend themselves to this kind of scrutiny. Generally, the less likely that a point, any point, in your form would seem for you to just stop cold, the more likely that your movement is at least influenced, if not driven, by momentum.

As mentioned earlier, under the right circumstances momentum can be a valuable and necessary part of your technique. The key to distinguishing between appropriate and inappropriate momentum lies in how the clarity of your *attention* and your *intention* is expressed via the movements of your body. As long as your momentum is deliberate and enhances your technique—whether in form practice, Push Hands with a partner, or in actual self defense application—there is no reason why it should not remain congruent with your overall goals at T'ai Chi.

Momentum in Class

Another consideration that you as a T'ai Chi student, and even more so if you are a teacher, may want to stay aware of is the momentum of any given class format or manner of teaching. Naturally, different teachers have different ways of presenting material and working with students. But if the classes you attend, or conduct, follow more or less the same predictable pattern class after class then the chances are that your classes are predicated at least somewhat on momentum. There is nothing inherently wrong with this, no more so than with any other occurrence of momentum, as long as you are aware of it and don't get stuck there. You might want to get in the habit, though, of occasionally asking yourself if your needs, or the ongoing needs of your students, are being well met by this approach?

I recognize my propensity as a teacher to count on a certain momentum when conducting group sessions. For the most part, I deem this an appropriate means of providing the group with the best instruction in meeting a range of students' needs. However, I also take pains to avoid getting stuck in any particular training approach by varying the curriculum and by scheduling special classes for the purpose of indulging myself and my students the opportunity to linger over this move, skill, concept, or that. Lingering and momentum are mutually exclusive dynamics; yet lingering is often just what students need in order to really grasp certain techniques or concepts.

Momentum of Your Mind

I would be remiss in covering this topic if I neglected to at least introduce the concept of momentum as a dynamic of the mind. The first seed of an idea for writing about momentum occurred to me as I was advising a student to beware the inappropriate momentum he displayed while demonstrating his form. I thought, "Hmm, I'll bet it would be great for readers if I could put together a short essay on this topic." I was thinking perhaps five hundred words, or so, my minimum for a short essay. As it turned out, the more I wrote about momentum the more my writing was taken over by the very quality I was writing about. Five hundred words stretched to a thousand, and then to twice that. It dawned on me as I wrote just how pervasive momentum is as an inadvertent and unconscious dynamic in the way people practice their T'ai Chi, whether in T'ai Chi form practice or in its other manifestations. For all the aforementioned reasons, momentum can be problematic as a physical dynamic, but also as a mental and psychological impediment to both your practice and to living your Tai Chi. Naturally, just as your mind and body mirror each other in so many other ways, so will they mirror each other in any tendency toward momentum. In order to effectively manage the momentum of your body during T'ai Chi, you must also pay attention for any tendency toward mental or emotional momentum.

How many times have you (or someone you've known) raced to class, still burdened with the concerns of your day, only to enter into a given round of form practice with a preconceived agenda already in place? "I will allot x amount of time for practice," or "I hope we practice in such and such a way, or focus on this or that, that I really enjoy," or "I hope we don't spend too much time in that stance that really fries my muscles." Mind you, having a well-organized agenda, one that you proceed to carry out deliberately, and even with momentum, is not inherently bad. But there can be an inertial downside to this as well. Some people get so invested in the momentum of their agenda that they forfeit their capacity for spontaneity. Instead, they find solace and safety in their momentum to an extent that it prevents them from truly settling themselves into the moment at hand.

Even more so than with your body, momentum can be problematic for your mind. Body momentum, when properly applied, can be a reliable and useful tool. Mental momentum, on the other hand, is much harder to keep in check, often manifesting as a loss of self-control. By mental momentum, I do not mean progressions of mental processes, such as I described above in relating how this chapter came to be. Nor do I mean to indict the implementation of strategies or ideas that may be well thought out and which may also have a constructive progression to them. I'm thinking rather of the kind of momentum that leads people to get carried away with themselves, that precludes clear and rational thinking, and which may be compensatory and premised on irrational reasoning, fixations, or emotional imbalances or insecurities. Or even just the momentum that carries us through our daily lives in the absence of any focused and deliberate attention to our own processes as they unfold.

Ironically, ineffectual momentum of the mind can occur as one consequence of being "stuck," or fixated on certain beliefs or premises. Just as is the case with your body, the propriety of mental momentum depends on the clarity of your intent and the quality of your attention.

Recognizing and reigning in inappropriate mental momentum, whether during T'ai Chi practice or at any other time, can work the same way with your mind as I described earlier regarding your body. Try to slow down or cease and desist with mental chatter and notice where this is difficult, versus where it is easy to do so. Any difficulty in "stepping back" and slowing down may indicate inappropriate momentum. You can experiment with managing mental momentum, just as you did earlier with body momentum, during T'ai Chi practice, or most especially during meditation, or whenever the notion occurs to you during your day.

In sum, momentum may be an unavoidable fact of life, but the key to using momentum wisely in T'ai Chi, or in life, is to not let it take precedence over other aspects. Toward this end, you want to remain as best you can attentive and intentive at all times.

CHAPTER 8

The Three Treasures Guide to Proper Stepping in T'ai Chi

I had fun selecting the title for this chapter. It sounds so classically sagacious. How sagacious this actually turns out to be will be up to you once you have completed this section and tried applying it to your own practice. The truth is it doesn't take a sage to figure out how to step properly. It all boils down to body mechanics.

As I see it, of all the important considerations to be factored into any step, whether you step forward or backward, there are three variables of primary concern. These considerations amount to nothing more than the three supporting joint areas of your lower body, which include your foot/ankle arrangement, your knee, and your *kua*. For the purposes of this discussion, we will regard your *kua* as including and governing your hips, waist, and tailbone. To keep this discussion simple, I will confine my description to forward stepping only. Once you have a grasp of the concepts in this chapter, you can apply them as you see fit to stepping patterns other than forward stepping.

Advancing forward from one stance into another is one of our most fundamental progressions in T'ai Chi. Simple T'ai Chi stepping is a skill that most practitioners have experimented with at some point in their training. Stepping forward is a necessary and unavoidable component of the great majority of techniques that occur in any T'ai Chi form, regardless of the style in question. Even when you only use your legs to move from one stance forward into the next—never mind what your upper body is doing—your advance would be as subject to the dictates of T'ai Chi principles as any of T'ai Chi's more complex whole body patterns. In order to step correctly, you must remain attentive to the full range of T'ai Chi's more global qualities, rooting and posture foremost among them. But, T'ai Chi's more encompassing qualities aside, the correctness of your stepping hinges, quite literally, on aligning your body in just the correct way at your supporting joints—your feet and ankles, your knees, and your *kua*/hips. To a lesser extent, certain of your middle and upper body joint areas come into play as well when stepping.

As a rule, how correct any technique is depends on the supporting joints below. In other words, your feet and ankles must be correct before your knees can be correct. And your knees must be correct, first, in order to properly align your *kua* and waist. Each joint's alignment and stability is premised on the joints supporting from below. It would seem to make the most sense then to start from below at the lowest point and work your way up, joint by joint, to insure that your body remains properly aligned at all times. You can now position yourself in a forward leaning stance and begin by looking down at your front foot and ankle, because that is where we will begin our exploration.

Turn Your Foot to Open the Door

I described the essential features and offered detailed instructions for basic T'ai

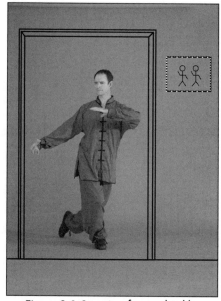

Figure 8-1 Stepping forward is like passing through a doorway.

Chi stepping in my first book, *Inside Tai Chi* (Loupos 2002) so I needn't repeat that full description here. But it will behoove you to recall the first (of several) most important points I made: in preparation for lifting your back leg and foot prior to stepping forward, you must first lift your toes and turn your front foot, angling it outward.

Each time you step forward your advance should be like passing through a doorway into your next stance (Figure 8-1). Prior to passing through the doorway, you must turn the doorknob to open the door. Opening your foot is akin to turning the door knob as it creates an opening, or channel, through which the rest of your body can pass. Turning your foot actually amounts to one of T'ai Chi's simplest moves. Turning your foot is neither complex, nor is it physically demanding. It is, however, essential and, judging from much of the T'ai Chi I have witnessed, fairly easy to neglect. Despite its ease, turning the front foot out prior to stepping is one of T'ai Chi's most oft forgotten details. The widespread negligence in turning the foot prior to stepping stems from the forward momentum that most people inadvertently rely on in advancing from stance to stance. I addressed momentum in some detail in the previous chapter, so I won't dwell on the topic here. In brief, inappropriate forward momentum provides a disincentive for practitioners to make the effort necessary to sink their weight back onto their rear foot prior to turning their front foot. Sinking back *first* is what should enable you to turn your front foot out with ease prior to shifting forward so you can glide

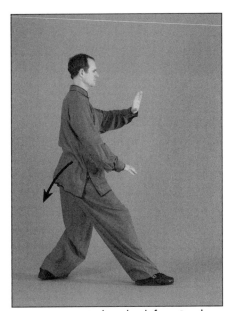

Figure 8-2. Sinking back from Brush Knee in preparation to advance.

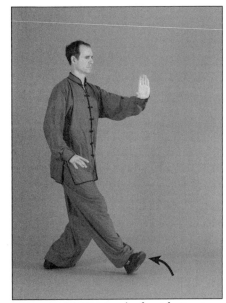

Figure 8-3 Turning the front foot out.

through the door. If you don't first sink back you cannot easily turn your front foot. And if you don't turn your foot you cannot turn your knee, and so on.

Turning your front foot is, thus, your first order of business. Assuming you are in a forward leaning stance, all you need do is sink your tailbone back toward your rear foot (Figure 8-2). Once you have sunk back, you can turn your front foot/ankle outward by forty-five degrees or so, according to your preference. You may need to experiment with this to find the angle that suits you best (Figure 8-3). Plant your foot flat and prepare to shift forward. That's all there is to it.

It is a curious anomaly that students seem always to remember to turn their foot out during T'ai Chi stepping when such turning is a specifically emphasized part of their assignment, such as during drill practice. Yet, they subsequently neglect to turn their foot out when their attention is more globally focused during form practice. I suspect this is because drill practices are inherently more repetitive and detail oriented. Anytime you practice the same move over and over, the tendency is to pay closer attention to each component of your move as it compares to the same move immediately preceding. Of course, this is why repetitive drill practices are employed in the first place, to give you the opportunity for such scrutiny. By contrast, it is easy to relapse and neglect certain details when practicing your form in its entirety. It is quite natural, if incorrect, to get caught up in the momentum of your form in its larger context and lose sight of the minutia. Nevertheless, you must remember to turn your front toes out prior to stepping forward if you wish to maintain a structural basis throughout.

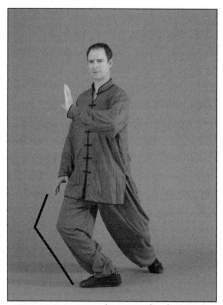

Figure 8-4a Knee bent too far forward.

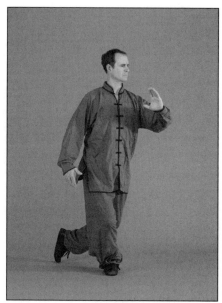

Figure 8-4b Knee correctly flexed over the toes.

Aligning Your Knee

Your second big concern is keeping your knee aimed correctly in relation to the foot below. The key here simply is to point your knee in the same direction as its foot, keeping it aligned throughout your step. To do otherwise compromises your knee structure and, by extension, the structure of everything above it. The degree to which you actually flex your knee varies from having it bent fully forward over your toes prior to sinking back, to having it completely straight once you have sunk back in preparation to turn your foot, to bending it again as you begin to shift your weight forward. Regardless of the degree of flex, take care to maintain your knee as aimed in the same direction that your foot is pointing. Also, try to avoid overbending your knee beyond the toes (Figures 8-4a and b). Finally, you want to avoid angling your knee either to the inside or to the outside of your foot (Figures 8-5a, b, and c). Any of these errors weaken the stability of your stance, at the least, and in the case of lateral misalignment you may actually jeopardize the stability and safety of the knee joint itself.

Thus far, the theory and the guidance for how to arrange your foot and your knee are fairly simple and straight forward. As unchallenging as all this may seem, these details are critical in laying a foundation for your next consideration, opening and aligning your *kua*.

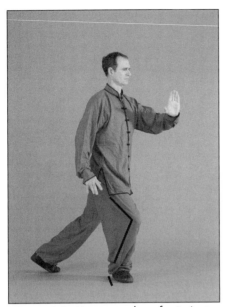

Figure 8-5a Knee turned too far in (note oblique angle of foot).

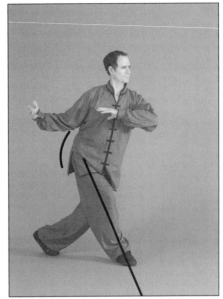

Figure 8-5b Knee turned too far out.

Opening Your *Kua* to Pass through the Door

Your third most important consideration in stepping forward is your *kua*, the location of which is indicated on either side of your centerline by your inguinal crease (Figure 8-6). In previous writings (Loupos 2002, 91-92), I noted the pivotal role of the *kua* in facilitating smooth and fluid movement throughout your form. I have especially noted the (correct) role of the *kua* in curbing the usual Beginners' tendency to bounce during transitions (Loupos 2002, 83-89).

Arranging your *kua* "just so" during T'ai Chi is so important that I find myself emphasizing and reemphasizing this connection for my own students throughout their studies. The challenge of imple-

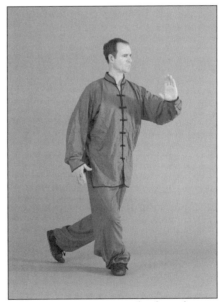

Figure 8-5c Knee correctly aligned over the foot.

menting this connection into your practice is underscored by the fact that these reminders to keep the *kua* open are as often directed at my more experienced students as toward students newer to T'ai Chi. In fact, after all my years of teaching, it still amazes me how challenging it can be for students to display a practical grasp of their *kua* connection despite regular and repeated reminders. By the intermediate level, students ought to be able to flow through their T'ai Chi with a familiar ease, as if it were a first or at least a second language. Yet some students find themselves mired in faulty practice patterns, which are more often than not exacerbated by their *kua* failing to articulate freely. There are few impediments as compromising to good T'ai Chi as that of an obstructed *kua*.

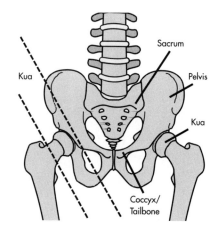

Figure 8-6 The kua, generally regarded as the loin/groin area, refers specifically to the inguinal crease.

For all the hoopla I make over this issue it might seem surprising when I say that learning the technique of *how* to open your *kua* is usually a breeze and painless. Most students, when shown how, are quick to grasp the theoretical benefits of maintaining an open *kua*. As a rule, I need only adjust a student's body to demonstrate how marked an improvement can be achieved at balance and rooting with the *kua* open versus closed. This never fails to elicit an enthusiastic nodding of the head. Even so, students regularly display difficulty in then integrating this new information into their form practice.

Naturally, there is an explanation for this. As important, and apparently simple, as opening the *kua* is, its positioning only exists in relation to other body parts. Any (re)arrangement of any part of your body must factor in all the other parts in order for T'ai Chi to be T'ai Chi. Your *kua* is no exception. The relative openness with which your *kua* is maintained must also take into account other body parts, and particularly those parts that are lower and closer to the earth, notably the knee below, and the foot below it. Clearly, if you are remiss in opening your foot prior to stepping, or in aligning your knee over that foot, you will have a poor foundation and little incentive to open the *kua*.

Assuming you have an adequate grasp of turning your foot and aligning your knee, let us proceed to examine the positioning of your *kua* more closely. We will start by examining that juncture point in your practice that is most critical in your transition from one stance to the next. If you can comprehend this then you earn an *A* in *kua*.

Your Most Elusive *Kua* Connection

The single most precarious point in stepping occurs just at the cusp of your attempt to shift the totality of your weight off one foot and onto the other, just as

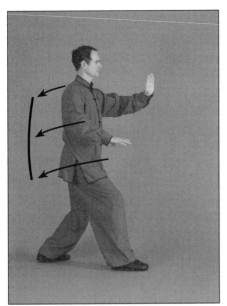

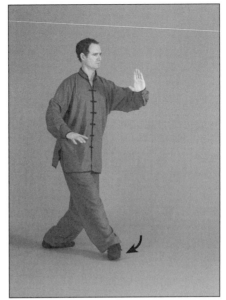

Figure 8-7a Sunk back from Brush Knee.

Figure 8-7b Toe out.

one foot becomes completely empty and the other foot becomes completely full. This cusp represents that point of transition I referred to earlier as "passing though the doorway." To best illustrate this connection the accompanying photos depict a generic advance for the lower body from one forward leaning stance into the next. Once you've got a generic grasp of this connection, you can apply its principles to any of your stance transitions.

Figures 8-7a, through 8-7e depict a stepping sequence. Figure 8-7a is included to provide a frame of reference only and may be disregarded once you are able to visualize the sequence. Our real concern is what happens between Figure 8-7c and Figure 8-7e. In Figure 8-7b, the subject has shifted forward to a point that his back leg is straight and much of his weight has been transferred to the front foot. Note that his back foot remains nearly flat at this point. In Figure 8-7d, his back heel is shown having peeled up as he has shifted additional weight forward onto the front foot. In Figure 8-7e, the transfer of weight from the back foot to the front foot is complete. In our next series of photographs, we will be examining the role of the *kua* in this transition.

You may want to engage the assistance of a partner for the directions that follow. Starting from the position shown Figure 8-7b, have your partner lean into one side of your *kua* and then the other (Figures 8-8a and b). Each side of your *kua* should be open and full so that the force of your partner's lean is transferred down through the same side foot to the earth. It is important that the force be transferred through the *same-side* foot. If either side of your *kua* collapses under duress (Figures

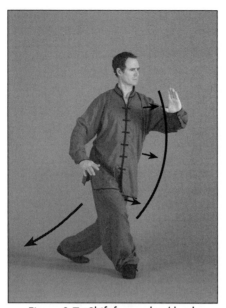

Figure 8-7c Shift forward w/ back
leg straight.

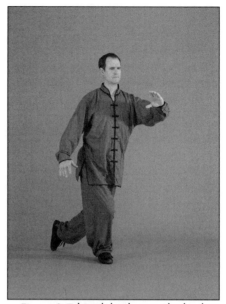

Figure 8-7d Back heel up as the back
knee flexes.

8-9a and b), you will need to take corrective measures to adjust your waist and
hips for stability before continuing on.
Proceed into the position shown in
Figure 8-7d, and again have your partner
lean into either side of your *kua*. To prevent collapse be careful to keep your tailbone curled under, as if your tailbone
were pressing your *kua* from behind to
encourage it open it a bit further. The
force of your partner's lean should continue to transfer down to your same-side
foot (Figures 8-10a and b).

We have now arrived at the most critical juncture point. As you proceed to
shift your weight completely off your
back foot and onto your front foot, again
with your partner leaning into first one
side of your *kua* and then the other, pay

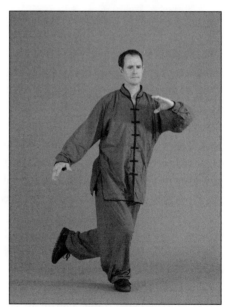

Figure 8-7e Back heel
becomes weightless.

close attention to where the force travels. On your more forward side (right in this
case), your partner's force should still transfer down through to the same (right-

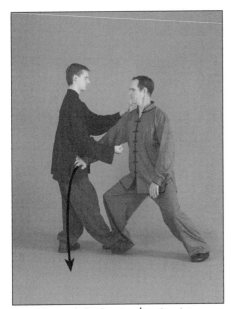

Figure 8-8a Partner leaning into the right kua . . .

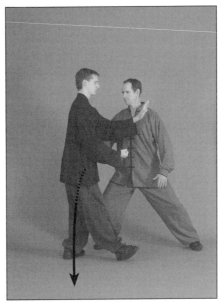

Figure 8-8b . . . and the left kua.

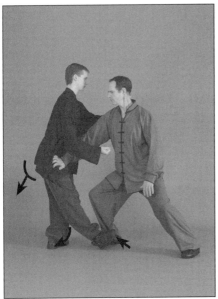

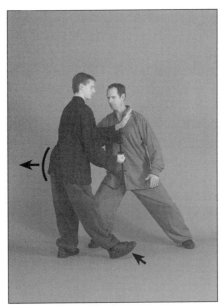

Figures 8-9a and b Don't let your kua collapse like this.

side) foot (Figure 8-11a). However, the force of his lean into your left-side *kua* should now transfer, as well, down to your right-side foot instead of to the same side left foot (Figure 8-11b).

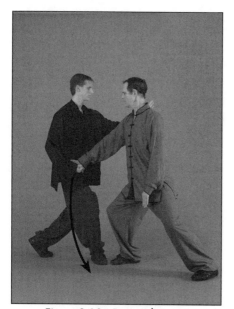

Figure 8-10a Partner leaning into the right kua . . .

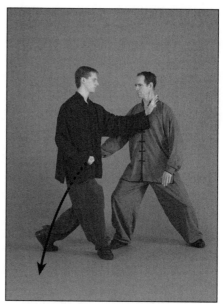

Figure 8-10b . . . and the left kua.

You need to pay attention, just prior to picking up your rear foot, for the place where your connection to the earth through that foot ceases to exist due to its *becoming empty*. It is exactly at that juncture point, where your weight and your partner's force shifts in its entirety from your rear foot to your front that you must scrutinize closely to insure that you never lose your feeling of connection to the earth. For most practitioners their transition through this juncture point is flawed due to their inadvertent reliance on momentum to carry them "through the doorway." You can easily determine whether you are carrying out this transition based on solid structure or compensatory momentum by having your partner lean against your *kua*, one side at a time, throughout your move. You must keep each side of your *kua* open and connected down through its corresponding foot until you transition fully onto your front foot (Figures 8-12a and b). Once you have gotten the feeling of this connection, your T'ai Chi is sure to feel steadier and more deeply rooted overall, as well as smoother and more fluid throughout.

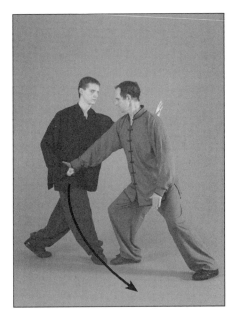

Figure 8-11a Partner's force goes through the right side to the right-side foot.

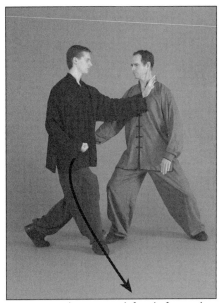

Figure 8-11b Partner's left-side force also goes through the right-side foot.

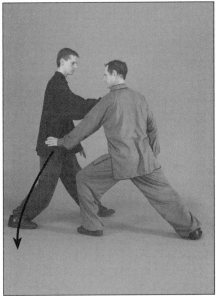

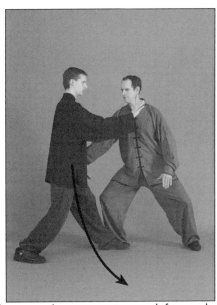

Figures 8-12a and b Keep your kua open and connected as you continue to shift toward conclusion of the move.

PART 3

Other Topics and Lectures

CHAPTER 9

Optimizing Your T'ai Chi Practice

Clearly, there are different styles of T'ai Chi. Also, different teachers who offer instruction in the same style often ascribe to different teaching methods. Even if you have only studied one way with one teacher, you need not always stay locked into practicing your T'ai Chi in just the way that you have learned it. This chapter explores a number of different approaches you can experiment with in varying the ways you practice and experience whatever T'ai Chi style or routine you are already accustomed to in order to provide you a more well-rounded experience.

Size Counts

Some styles of T'ai Chi offer different interpretations, or versions of T'ai Chi within the context of that style. For example, there are "large frame" and also "small frame" variations in some styles. A large frame version of T'ai Chi emphasizes larger and more expansive movements, while the smaller frame variations offer a more condensed positioning and movement. As a rule, larger frame versions are regarded as training fodder for students newer at T'ai Chi. Progressively smaller frame versions may be indicated for students as their skill level improves over time.

The advantage of smaller frame versions is that everything about your practice tends to remain more consolidated, and therefore more potentially explosive. The practitioner will be much more likely to develop an awareness of and a sensitivity to where his body is at any given time, in terms of how the body's different components interact and engage. This makes sense because when separate body components work together in a more contained proximity, they tend to be more tightly knit, more intraconnected as well as interconnected.

With the larger frame version, your body spreads itself out more. Larger frame versions are more appropriate for beginners because the scale of the movement requires relatively less of the precision so necessary in a more tightly knit movement pattern. Hence, the intraconnection dilutes somewhat as your body opens itself up. You enjoy a greater extension and range of motion, along with the challenge of keeping your body properly engaged even as it is fully expanded. Acquiring this kind of skill can be challenging to the extent that body parts that are distanced further apart still need to move with precise synchronization.

As noted, some T'ai Chi styles have a framework hierarchy built into their systems of practice. Others pay this distinction little (apparent) heed. If the style in which you train does not offer variable contexts, you may benefit from experimenting on your own and within your existing practice context. In other words, you can vary the manner in which you practice whatever T'ai Chi you already do to make it larger or smaller. Practice variations such as this are inadvisable for novice and beginner level students. More advanced students who are already familiar with minimalization of movements and the subtleties of connections therein may find benefit, even if just comparative, by trying to apply the qualities of nuance to a larger frame variation. With practice, you'll find yourself able to apply the nuances of the smaller context to the larger version without compromising the natural essence of the small.

Generally, it is advisable for students to learn a particular way of practicing T'ai Chi and then try to improve their skills within the context of that practice. This can become problematic, though, if students get so locked into that context that their practice methods fail to evolve and develop along with their general skill levels. When students become locked in, so to speak, they run the risk of creating their own rigid patterns. Please don't misconstrue what I'm recommending as a dismissal of traditional values or training methods. Lest I give the impression that I am cavalier about adhering to traditional values, let me emphasize that I recognize that there is a great deal of information and knowledge latent in any traditional T'ai Chi system. This information and knowledge can take years or even decades to decipher fully. I am not of the opinion that students should be pretentious in disregarding the untapped potential of their existing practice material in favor of some more novel approach simply for the sake of novelty. But, under a skilled teacher's supervision, or if you are already quite skilled on your own, you can realize an even higher level of proficiency for yourself by experimenting with the "relative scale" of your usual form routine.

Move Slow, Move Fast

You can also experiment with varying the pace of your practice. T'ai Chi is usually practiced slowly, but slowness is relative in any case. You might try decelerating your form (so that it requires more practice time) by increments of several minutes at a time, assuming you practice the long form, or by smaller increments if you practice a shorter version, such as the 24-move form. When you opt to experiment with a slower pace, be attentive to the quality (internal nuances) as well as the quantity (actual pace) of your form. Previously (chapter 1), I discussed the idea of opportunities in slowness. Of the many variables discussed, most are themselves subject to adjustment and variation according to just how slow you go.

During any relatively faster version of your practice, be sure to pay special heed to your body's larger joints, both for safety and for special readjustments. Also, you will find that adding pace to your form will challenge the ability of your muscles to keep all the different parts of your body coordinated and to keep you flowing smoothly from your center. This will be especially so over the course of any prolonged practice session as your muscles inevitably fatigue.

Be Soft

In addition to experimenting with the pace of your form, you might also try varying the amount of force you employ. T'ai Chi is generally regarded as being "soft" but this, of course, is a relative quality just like any other. During any given practice session, the softness with which you execute your moves can vary considerably. This may happen naturally in reflection of your mood or your energy level, whether emotional, mental, or physical, or you may deliberately adjust your level of softness, or lack thereof, according to a predetermined agenda.

In all likelihood, you already have a certain standard quality of softness commensurate with your ability with which you normally carry out your practice. You can depart from that standard by trying to relax and soften your moves even more so than usual. The list that follows contains a number of suggestions for how you can soften your practice. In each case, try to apply the given suggestion with your hands first as your hands quite naturally command your attention due to their leading role in most movements. Then use that feeling of more relaxed softness in your hands as a model, or cue, for softening the rest of your movement.

1. Try breathing through the pores of your skin into your bones.
2. Try to expand and elasticize your joints.
3. Feel yourself displacing, minimally, the air you move through.
4. "Listen" with your hands.
5. Let your hands flow through the air in the lightest possible way.

Bring Your Power to the Surface

Softness and power are not mutually exclusive features. It is possible for you to have and to express both these qualities in your T'ai Chi. Most practitioners are aware, even if not through their own direct personal experience, that T'ai Chi has the potential for great expressions of power, as in its fabled *fa jin* force. But few practitioners attain, or even come near to attaining, real T'ai Chi power. There seems to be a widespread presumption that practicing slowly and softly will eventually, and somehow automatically, lead to great power and speed as resources in one's practice. Not so. Slowness and softness merely set the stage so that you can then proceed to develop power and speed in a manner congruent with T'ai Chi principles. The development of real power and real speed happens only after you have developed a body that is able to move fluidly and from your center. Learn to

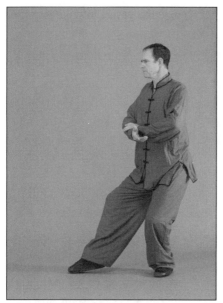

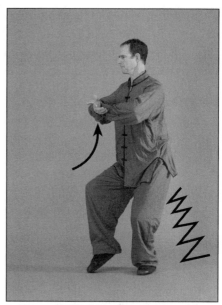

Figure 9-1 Hands in the ready position, preparing to Press.

Figure 9-2 Raising the arms up while sinking the weight back onto the rear foot.

move your body with efficiency first through slowness and softness. Then you have a basis for learning how to move with power and speed. The gulf between slowness/softness and power/speed is no short span. Years of practice may be required before you achieve a reasonable command of these more advanced skills.

That said, you can begin to get a feel for how to incorporate power and speed into your practice by experimenting with the following training methods. Beware, though, to keep your ambition in check. If this kind of exercise is premature for you at your current level of training, you may accomplish little more than reinforcing bad habits, such as overreliance on strength and muscular force, usually referred to as *li*. Or, if you overdo it, you may cause yourself harm due to overuse of weak muscles or as a consequence of poor body structure.

Nearly any move or posture can be adapted to the drill that follows. I will use the move Press as an example to get you started, and then you can experiment from there on your own. Prepare to begin as shown in Figure 9-1. Raise your arms as you gather earth force up from below and set back just a bit (loading up) onto your rear foot (Figure 9-2). Next, raise your front knee and round your body as you prepare to issue force. A timely caveat here is to avoid any tendency to "wind up" in your lower back (Figure 9-3). Despite the whiplike feeling that may accompany winding up, this will only dilute the power you are able to deliver toward your target. Instead, keep your lower back full (Figure 9-4) and drive from your legs and waist. Step out forward with your front leg while keeping your upper body connected to your lower body though your waist and tailbone (Figure 9-5). As you plant into

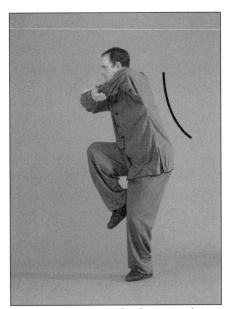

Figure 9-3 Lower back incorrectly cocked back, or wound up, prior to releasing force.

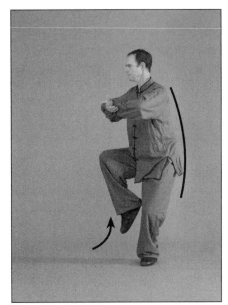

Figure 9-4 Front knee raised and body rounded in preparation to drive from legs and waist.

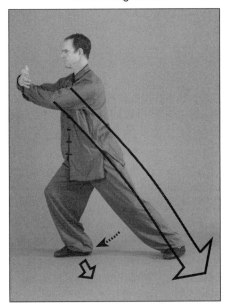

Figure 9-5 Front leg steps forward and roots.

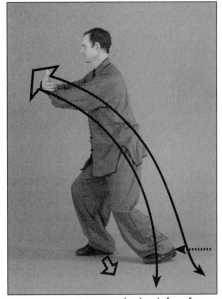

Figure 9-6 Bringing the back foot forward while pressing out.

your front leg, drag/push your back foot along from behind to amplify the issuance of your pressing force (Figure 9-6). Repeat this technique as many times as you like while advancing forward along a straight line. Then turn around and practice the opposite side going back in the other direction.

The more times you practice this, the more familiar you will become with the move. Repetition breeds familiarity, and familiarity will promote sensitivity to the subtle nuances necessary to gain real skill. You can adapt almost any T'ai Chi move to some similar sort of a skill development drill pattern. However you choose to apply your creative skills to whatever moves you deem suitable for practice, be sure to start slowly so that you can feel your internal connections *prior* to emphasizing speed or force. Only when you are sure of your connections, should try to add pace and power.

Shake to Your Root

Another way you can improve your T'ai Chi is by vibrating yourself through your form as a way to feel your body connected and rooted. The best way for me to explain this approach is to draw on the example of tall buildings that have been built to resist damage by earthquakes. Instead of having foundations that are rigid and unyielding these buildings have enormous springs built into their foundations as shock absorbers. These springs allow the buildings to rock a bit when the earth rolls. No matter how the earth quakes, these buildings just roll with the punches. You too can benefit through feeling yourself as if rooted onto shock absorbers.

Stationary shaking and vibrating in one form or another is something I have known all my most skilled teachers to rely on, either for its benefits as a healing method or as a means of loosening the body, both physically and energetically. Stationary shaking is a standard element in my pre-class warm up routines. I also like to make shaking, or its subtler expression as a shiverlike vibration, an occasional part of my moving practice. Every now and then during form practice, I'll practice vibrating my whole body, not in a continuous nonstop manner, but as a means of occasionally checking and challenging my root and my body alignment. When I do this, the vibration in my legs reinforces my root, as if I am preparing to launch an attack off either leg. You may also notice places in your body that fail to shake or vibrate freely due to tightness, stagnation, or stress. Identifying problems areas is the first step in implementing corrective measures. Vibrating through your form will help you attune to your body and free yourself of tension all at once.

As is the case with so many T'ai Chi drills and skills, vibrating also lends itself to partner work. For example, if you position yourself in a forward leaning stance, you can practice vibrating both of your legs from front to back, as if you were trying to fix your feet more firmly down to the floor. While vibrating, ask a partner to first pull against your front knee, and then push. Then your partner can move around behind you and try pushing and pulling against your back knee. In each case your stance should remain firmly attached, rooted, to the floor below. As always when it comes to knees, take care not to use undue force: Remember to put safety first.

External Variables

In most cases the variables with which you will be concerned are internal: shaking, power, range of movement, etc. However, the environmental conditions under which you practice can also have an effect on your experience during any given practice session.

One important consideration may be whether your practice is indoors or outdoors. For example, if you are indoors what type of flooring do practice on? Carpet, wood, and concrete vary in the support and traction they afford you. Over the long term, flooring surfaces can also have an impact on your ankles, knees, and back.

If you practice outside, is quite possible that the weather and temperature conditions under which you practice are a consideration. There are few experiences I enjoy more than starting out on a warm, sunny spring morning with some pondside T'ai Chi practice. However, I live in New England, so spring is but a passing fancy and weather conditions tend to be fickle. I have been known to practice on my pond when it is frozen solid with just a frosting of snow, but generally I'm disinclined to practice on snow or ice. Outdoors practice can also be affected by your terrain. Lawns, beaches, parking lots, rooftops, and uneven surfaces all have their own unique feel and challenge to them.

If your practice is indoors, the quality of lighting, or absence thereof, may be a consideration. Also, the time of day or night that you practice, the amount of time that you allot for your training sessions, and even the air quality all have some impact on your experience. You may not be able to tinker with all these variables in the same manner as your more internal conditions, but just being aware of them can help to insure that your attunement with your practice environment remains harmonious. Any or all of these considerations can influence your subjective experience (a la *feng shui*) in how you are able to blend in or feel attuned to your immediate surroundings. The effect and the value of these considerations should not be underestimated.

Along with flooring conditions and external environments is the issue of footwear, or the absence thereof. Bare feet, sandals, T'ai Chi shoes, or army boots will each influence your practice, again depending on your flooring surface, in ways that can surprise and delight or frustrate and detract.

Now that you have invested as much time and energy into getting your T'ai Chi just as close to perfect as you and your teacher might hope for, it may seem that I have given you license to rewrite all the rules. Not so; well not exactly. I'm not suggesting that you abandon or replace any of what you've striven to accomplish in the past. I am suggesting that you play with the ideas in this chapter to continually challenge yourself by constantly (or even just occasionally) questioning and testing the limits of your T'ai Chi. Whether you experiment with frame size, velocity, shaking, power moves, or T'ai Chi at the beach, your open and questioning mind will renew the freshness of your learning experience and keep you from becoming stuck in complacency.

CHAPTER 10

Other Lectures

Integrating T'ai Chi into Other Martial Arts Programs

It delights me no end to report that the mainstream martial arts community here in the United States is finally starting to give T'ai Chi Ch'uan its due recognition. I wish I could credit this community with recognizing T'ai Chi on its merits, but the fact is that this recognition is consumer-based. By this I mean that enough consumers have, on their own, taken an interest in T'ai Chi to cause harder style school owners to sit up and take notice, or risk being left out of the game. Just as with the earlier aerobics, kickboxing, and Tae Bo fads school owners are anxious to position themselves early on so as not to miss out. Indeed, T'ai Chi has all the potential to be a lucrative addition to any school's martial arts program. Furthermore, T'ai Chi is here to stay and unlikely to succumb to fickle market tastes as so often happens with other fads.

But there is a rub. In order to be "well positioned" teachers have three choices, as I see it: 1) they can teach T'ai Chi themselves, *which means they have to learn it first*; 2) they can hire someone who is already skilled at T'ai Chi to do their teaching for them; or 3) they can decide that options 1 and 2 are inconvenient, for whatever reasons, and convince themselves that a gullible public can easily be hood-winked into believing that any slowed down version of martial arts amounts to real T'ai Chi. Option 3 is the "low road" and clearly unacceptable for anyone who values integrity and a good reputation in the community.

I will emphasize right off that I am not a proponent of any attempt to propagate T'ai Chi solely for its potential as an exploitable resource. The last thing I want is to see T'ai Chi being treated like the next lucrative fad. The reality, however, is that T'ai Chi's popularity is growing by leaps and bounds, and where there is a demand a supply is sure to appear to meet that demand. What then is the best way to proceed?

Option 1 is just fine, except that exactly what is entailed in learning T'ai Chi may come as something of a shock to many harder style martial artists. T'ai Chi entails a much more comprehensive learning experience than many assume. Though it is quite true that harder style martial arts teachers may bring some skills with them, i.e., teaching skills, fitness, martial mindsets, body awareness, etc., it is just as true that those skills are as likely to be liabilities as assets when it comes to

T'ai Chi. Undertaking a study of T'ai Chi is more akin to starting out again as a white belt than it is to taking a weekend seminar in kickboxing. So, what's an instructor to do? (More on your best approach shortly.)

There's always option 2. Hiring someone who is already qualified to teach may be your easiest solution. This arrangement will save you the time that would otherwise be necessary to develop actual skills at T'ai Chi for yourself. But how do you know that the person you hire is really qualified? If you think traditional Kung Fu is confusing without a built-in belt ranking system to indicate someone's skill level, T'ai Chi will try your patience. Traditionally, T'ai Chi eschews much of the structure and hierarchy that characterize harder style martial arts. Though it is not unheard of for T'ai Chi schools to have adopted a belt ranking system, this is by far the exception rather than the rule. Personally, I would be hard pressed to give serious consideration to any teaching candidate who told me he had a Black Belt in T'ai Chi Ch'uan. T'ai Chi teachers are usually pretty informal and many don't even require uniforms. So don't let yourself be automatically put off if a teaching candidate presents as more casual than formal. This might actually be a good sign.

If, on the other hand, you hire someone who is highly skilled at T'ai Chi, he or she may decide to go it alone after building a following in your school and you will be back to square one. These concerns aside, if you hire the right qualified teacher you may be on your way to a successful program. An arrangement such as this can work very well for some, but it won't be for everybody.

My great concern is that otherwise professional martial artists may forego options 1 or 2 in favor of 3. My apprehension here actually has less to do with out and out duplicity and more to do with ignorance. There are so many T'ai Chi video courses available that school owners could hardly be faulted for assuming that, "you learn to do these simple moves slowly and, presto, you know T'ai Chi." I have seen this happen and it's a real shame because, in the end, everybody loses. Wanna-be teachers who have done just this have also become the laughing stock among those more in the know.

> **Other style instructors who wish to add a T'ai Chi component to their curriculum must understand that there are no shortcuts involved in learning T'ai Chi. Know this: T'ai Chi cannot be learned to any level of real skill from a video or other media, period. The good news is that your learning process can be fast tracked, relatively speaking, by avoiding certain mistakes and pitfalls that might otherwise lead you astray, costing you time, money, and aggravation. Read on.**

As with any other learning endeavor, it pays to educate yourself first by learning as much as you can *about* your subject prior to committing to a course of study. With T'ai Chi the best way to do that is to sit in on classes that others are

teaching and/or to read as much as you can about the subject. The three books I
have authored to date were written with just this in mind and are guaranteed to
address many of the concerns you may have about learning and, eventually, teaching T'ai Chi. Other Tai Chi books or media may be comparably suited to this task.
You must also keep in mind that there are different styles of T'ai Chi as well as different teaching approaches ascribed to by different instructors. These different
styles or teaching methods will likely vary in the appeal they hold for you. So, educate yourself first, then shop around.

   You will also need to remember that you must be a student before you can be
a teacher. Just as all instructors expect this from their own students, so must you be
prepared to start at square one with T'ai Chi. Aside from whatever commercial
benefits you may be hoping to derive from offering T'ai Chi at your club or school,
T'ai Chi can complement and deepen your own understanding of whatever else
you are already skilled at. Investors in fine art are always advised to buy what they
like, so that they can live with it even if the market tanks. The same can be said for
T'ai Chi. Learn it for yourself first and don't rush into being a teacher.

   If you have a qualified T'ai Chi instructor in your area with whom you are
comfortable studying, fine. Otherwise you may have to travel. One good way to
expedite your own learning process is to participate in T'ai Chi seminars or camps,
many of which are suitable for entry level learners. You can find listings for seminars and camps posted on the internet or in the major T'ai Chi magazines. Another
excellent, and convenient, option is to "import" a teacher. A number of well qualified T'ai Chi teachers augment their regular teaching schedules by traveling to
teach at other schools. Quite a lot can be taught in the course of a day long or
weekend presentation. I take great pleasure in this myself because it is always
refreshing to share T'ai Chi with teaching colleagues and their students. With the
right marketing, this kind of arrangement can allow host instructors to "earn while
they learn." Of course, and not unreasonably, some instructors may be reticent
about putting themselves into a learning environment right alongside their own
students. A skilled guest teacher will be sensitive to these concerns and take steps
to insure that the host instructor retains "face" throughout the learning process.
Host instructors who have foresight, or who are particularly keen to learn, can even
arrange private lesson time for themselves to insure that they stay a few steps ahead
of their own students between seminars. Then, they will be in a position to conduct practice and review classes for their own students until, eventually, they are
qualified to assume the fuller helm of teaching responsibilities.

   However you plan to integrate T'ai Chi into your school's existing curriculum,
remember that T'ai Chi is not simply slowed down karate. T'ai Chi is a fully
autonomous martial art with a wide range of benefits for those engaged in its study.
If you make the commitment to "do it right" T'ai Chi will give you a big return on
your investment.

Discernment

One of the best lines in my second book, *Exploring Tai Chi*, was not written by me but by Dr. Jay Dunbar, who graciously authored the foreword to that text. Said Dr. Jay, "Tai Chi is an exercise in discernment. Expertise consists in being able to differentiate between subtly different situations and conditions."

How true! But how do you accomplish the ability to discern and differentiate between T'ai Chi's many subtleties? Simply put, you must repeat, review, and adjust accordingly. Then *repeat*, *review* and *adjust* all over again, and again, and again.

Your first and ongoing task is to repeat, or practice, that which you have learned. New learnings are almost always absorbed, initially, in their grossest and least detailed form. The more you repeat a move or a pattern the more thoroughly that pattern will become ingrained in your body/mind, and the less attention you will need to pay to recalling the move's grosser level details. As your pattern becomes more familiar through repetition, you will naturally develop an enhanced sensitivity to slight, and increasingly slighter, variations and nuances in how your move is performed.

Next then, once repetition has you feeling more confident about your practice, it is time for critical review. The constancy and rote of repetitive practice may, at times, seem to verge on automatic pilot, but critical review, as opposed to practice, will entail more emphasis on discernment. At this stage, it is no longer sufficient to merely notice variations in your practice. When you review your T'ai Chi material, you must do so with a regard to detail and also with the intention of comparative analysis. Now is the time to tap into your capacity for critical thinking as discussed in chapter 1 in order to compare ever more subtle variations in your practice, and sort through to determine the relative value of each variation in comparison to the others.

Theoretically, your adjustment stage would follow, and you would be tweaking here and shifting there and strengthening or softening in yet another place. Adjustment represents the more results-oriented phase in this trilogy. In this phase, you will not repeat moves only by rote, nor will you merely sense for subtle variations in your practice, you will actively experiment with them in a deliberate manner. Deliberately orchestrated variations might revolve around power, pacing, frame size, or other postural adjustments. Or, you might just work with natural variations as they occur in more subtle ways. Just as with the review process, you will become increasingly more exacting in your differentiations as you improve over time. As you might surmise, this stage remains closely intertwined with the review stage, as each small shift or variation that you experiment with will, in turn, be subject to its own review process. It may take a good bit of tinkering before your adjustments feel fully satisfactory in meeting the requirements for good T'ai Chi. In fact, you may (should) never reach a point in your training where complacency supplants perseverance. But, as noted by Dr. Jay, that's the nature of discernment and the path one must follow in order to accomplish real expertise at T'ai Chi.

Trick or Skill?

As a T'ai Chi teacher with roots tracing back several decades in the same community, I am often called upon to present on T'ai Chi to various groups. These audiences run the gamut from civic groups to corporate entities to young school children. I always relish activities such as these because they give me an opportunity to share with others something I care about very deeply. I take great pleasure in enlightening people who know very little about T'ai Chi, regard-

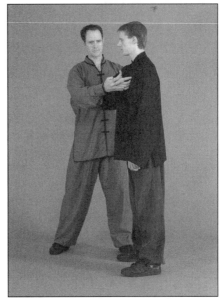

Figure 10-1 A big, strong volunteer.

less of whether they may be suitable candidates for its study, to the magic that T'ai Chi has to offer.

As much as I enjoy these kinds of presentations it is often the case that I am allotted only a limited amount of time in which to address my audience. In the time assigned, I must make my best effort to communicate the fundamental intricacies of T'ai Chi, as well as what it is about T'ai Chi that renders it so attractively unique in the vast field of mind and/or body personal development disciplines. And this in consideration that T'ai Chi, almost by definition, is anything but expeditious. Thus, I am challenged to make a good impression quickly and superficially about something which is inherently slow and profound.

As a rule, I do manage to keep it intriguing for those in attendance when I explain T'ai Chi theory and the many potential benefits that T'ai Chi holds for anyone who commits to regular and correct practice. But, what really grabs people's attention is when I engage the assistance of a couple of unwitting audience members to demonstrate just how plainly simple it can be to accomplish T'ai Chi body structure, and in a way that is clearly effective regardless of age, gender, body size, or muscle mass.

Usually, this entails starting with some big, strong looking volunteer whose predictable reliance on muscular resistance fails to withstand the duress of my slow but steady push (Figure 10-1). Following this, I ask for someone smaller and considerably less intimidating, ideally a small woman or child, to step up. A few minor adjustments in body positioning is all it usually takes to ensure that this person's

structure can adequately withstand whatever force I am about to apply (Figure 10-
2). The results of this experiment/
demonstration are clear in their message.
Audience members sit up and take notice
and can't help but smile or nod their
heads as they think to themselves, "I can
do that."

All I have really done to make my
point is to employ a few T'ai Chi "tricks"
to impress upon my viewers that anybody
can accomplish T'ai Chi structure and
rooting with the right guidance. Actually,
despite my tendency to ham it up just a
bit, "tricks" probably is not the best word
to describe what I do. A trick, after all, is
something other than what it appears to
be, often entailing some element of
deception or slight of hand. In truth,

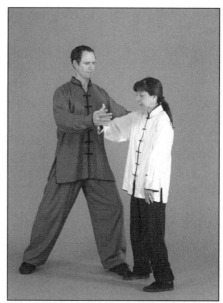

Figure 10-2 Applying force against a
well-structured subject.

what my volunteers and audience members are getting is their very first lesson at
T'ai Chi body alignment. The results that stem from the manipulation of my volunteers only *look* like tricks because most audience members are so far out of touch
with what their own bodies can accomplish.

People like to be tricked (hence the popularity of magic shows and movies featuring special effects). Tricksters are believed to hold some special skill or knowledge which those they entertain are not meant to be privy to. This is where my
presentation differs from that of mere entertainment, as I invite the audience inside
the trick. Even as contrived as are the outcomes of my demonstration scenarios,
audience members can feel themselves empowered just by witnessing the applied
principles of T'ai Chi body structure. As much as people like to be entertained,
they inevitably prefer to be empowered, in this case from learning how a few simple adjustments to their body can offer them a newfound source of personal
strength and power.

T'ai Chi skills only appear as tricks to those unschooled in their intricacies.
The difference between being tricked and being empowered can be as simple as
"being in" on how the trick or skill works. Therefore, the most important job of
the T'ai Chi teacher is just that—to get his or her students on the *inside* of how
T'ai Chi works so that students themselves become empowered through their practice and training. When you are on the inside it is very hard for anybody to pull
the wool over your eyes.

Extend, But Don't Reach

Oftentimes there are semantic nuances in the T'ai Chi learning process that are sufficiently discrepant as to mislead even the keenest students. One example of this is the difference between "extending" and "reaching."

How many times might you have heard your teacher advise, "Extend your arm," or "Extend your stepping foot?" But, when you execute your technique that advice somehow translates to "reach my arm out," or "now I must reach with my foot." This is an understandable mix-up as the difference in connotation between these two words, *extend* and *reach*, is quite subtle. In fact, in cross-checking for their definitions I noted that my dictionary uses each of these words as a synonym for the other. For general usage *reach* and *extend* are regarded as interchangeable terms. However, T'ai Chi can be an exacting discipline and, as such, often requires an exacting vocabulary to convey its intricacies.

The word *reach* conjures up in my mind a certain action. It implies action that is predicated on an amount of effort commensurate with that action. To "reach one's goal," or to "reach the end zone," or to "reach out and touch someone," or to "reach an agreement" are clichés that come to mind. None of these is particularly passive and all seem to imply not only the process but the end result of an effort made, as if inroads were realized in the face of resistance or challenge.

Extend, by comparison, conjures up something just slightly, yet significantly, different. To "extend one's self," or to "extend greetings," or to "extend an offer," or to "extend a courtesy" all seem a bit more passive. This word offers no suggestion of inroads having been achieved despite difficulty. Rather *extend* connotes a state of affairs somewhat less finalized than *reach*, a process within a process. *Extend* seems somehow less driven by a need for goal and more associated with an offer of opportunity in some form or another.

> Where *reach* is less concerned with the process of reaching than it is with the goal of what has been reached, *extend* is all about the process of extending and much less about the bottom line of having finally reached an end result. These nuances are not lost in T'ai Chi. When your teacher asks you to *extend* your arm he is likely much less concerned with where your arm ends up than with how it gets there.

When you reach with your arm, as if for some object, your goal is to grasp that object. You use your muscles to stretch your arm until that object has been reached. Reaching with your arm implies nothing beyond face value—your arm reaches. By comparison, when you extend your arm in T'ai Chi, its muscles may stretch, but your muscles are only a secondary concern. Extension as we emphasize it in T'ai Chi is much more about opening your joints and expanding from deeply within from your bones and tendons, and not just from the external musculature, nor even just

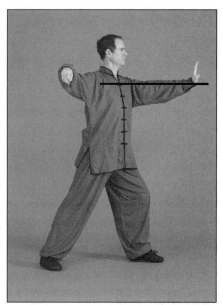 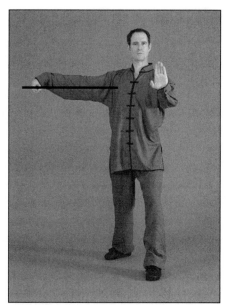

Figures 10-3a and b Arms "reaching" in Single Whip.

from your arm. Extending necessarily entails the involvement of your whole body, from your shoulder through your tailbone and so on down to the earth. You *extend* from your heart, or your center, whereas you *reach* from your arm socket. Reaching is unidirectional, whereas extending is multidirectional. More on this shortly.

By way of example, please refer to Figures 10-3a, b, and c where you see our subject shown in a Single Whip posture. In the first two photos (Figures 10-3a and b), he is reaching with both of his arms. In the third photo (Figure 10-3c), his arms are extended. In the first case, even though his lower body may be properly grounded, our subject is vulnerable to instability. Because reaching fails to take into account the rest of his body the integrity of the arm-to-body connection is compromised, and so is his root (Figures 10-4a through 10-4d). In comparison, by extending his arms our subject maintains their connection to the rest of his body, and ultimately to the earth (Figures 10-4e through 10-4h). Though our subject's arms are extended, so are his elbows, extending (setting) down toward the earth; so are his scapulae extending (expanding) away from one another; and so is his tailbone extending, down (a la *sung*), all with the purpose in mind of augmenting his rootedness.

The upshot is that reaching affords you extension, but at the expense of root because it precludes that T'ai Chi relaxation quality known as *sung*. Extending, on the other hand, allows you to reach, but without losing your whole body connection. Extending makes an allowance for that quality of *sung*. I'll talk more about *sung* in the next section. For now, though, try to experiment and feel the difference between reaching with your arm or your leg, versus extending.

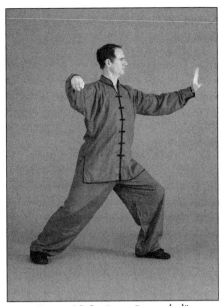

Figure 10-3c Arms "extended" in Single Whip.

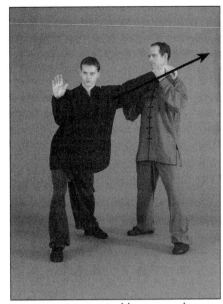

Figure 10-4a Unable to neutralize a pulling force...

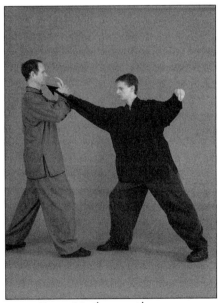

Figure 10-4b ...to either arm.

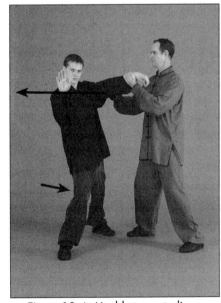

Figure 10-4c Unable to neutralize a pushing force...

Sink Back and Relax While We Discuss *Sung*

Sung is one of those elusive T'ai Chi concepts that fails to translate entirely satisfactorily into English. Usually, *sung* translates as relaxation. For practitioners who are already well-versed in the subtleties of this quality, interpreting *sung* to simply

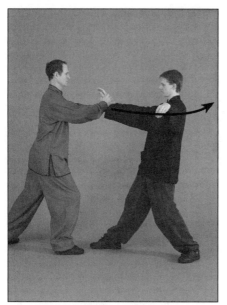

Figure 10-4d ...to either arm.

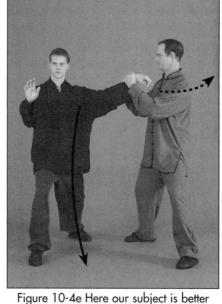

Figure 10-4e Here our subject is better able to transfer a pulling force through his arms and down to the earth.

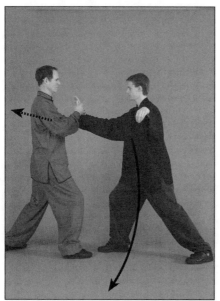

Figures 10-4f Neutralizing a pulling force from the front.

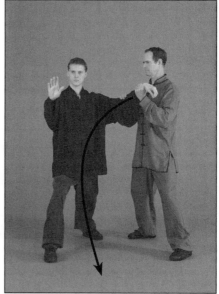

Figures 10-4g Neutralizing a pushing force from the side.

mean relaxation will suffice, but only because those already privy to the nuances of *sung* need no further elucidation on the subject. For students whose understanding and command of *sung* is less thorough and less conspicuous, simply calling *sung* relaxation is misleading, at best.

In our culture the idea of relaxation may conjure up anything from active recreation to kicking back on the couch. For some people taking a nap is relaxing. But that is not *sung*. For folks at the opposite end of the spectrum rock climbing may be relaxing. But that is still a far cry from *sung*. Either napping on the couch or rock climbing may be greatly enhanced by *sung*, but *sung* is not inherent to the activity.

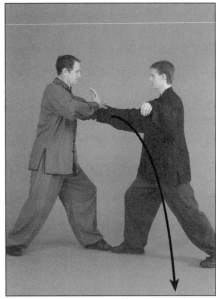

Figures 10-4h Neutralizing a pushing force from the front.

Sung implies relaxation, yes, but not limpness or flaccidity. With *sung* there is relaxation, but with a certain tensile continuity, as if there were strength present and available in the absence of work or effort being made. Here are three examples of ways you might think of *sung* in order to help you somatize this concept in your own body.

One way to think of *sung* is as if it were a chain that has been stretched and suspended between two points. No matter how tightly the chain has been stretched, there is still bound to be some sag at its midpoint. This settling at the midpoint can be thought of as *sung*. The chain, though fully stretched, is every bit as relaxed as it possibly can be under the circumstances, yet there is a latent force coursing through it that prevents its collapsing down further yet.

Another way you might think of *sung* is as a sponge cake. If you press down with your hand against a sponge cake, it compresses, yielding to your force. Yet, as soon as you remove your hand, the cake springs back up. Its softness is such that it will not resist your force, yet its resilience allows it to regain and retain its form.

Finally, you might think of *sung* as evident in a needle floating on water, or rather as one property of the water that supports the needle. Even though a needle made of steel is much heavier than water the tensile continuity of the water's surface, due to its surface tension, allows it to support the heavier object. As soft and as yielding as water is, the force with which it holds itself together precludes its collapse. You can think of your lower body, from your waist down, as being like water, the surface tension of which allows your upper body to settle into it, yet be supported from below.

Just as a chain sags at its center yet remains strong, or a sponge cake yields only to spring back and regain its form, or water holds itself together even while supporting a denser object, T'ai Chi practice encourages us to emulate nature's *sung*. Of course, this is easier said than accomplished. Most people carry a level of tension in their bodies that makes a consistent and effortless expression of *sung* challenging, at best. (For an explanation of impediments to accomplishing *sung*, refer to *Exploring Tai Chi* (Loupos 2003), chapter 3, "Trust and Surrender versus Cognition and Control.")

Let's refer back to our Single Whip photo from the previous section in which our subject has extended his arms (Figure 10-5). In this photo, you can see, as indi-

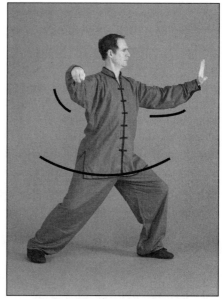

Figure 10-5 The subject's waist, shoulders and elbows are 'set', resilient but not drooping.

cated by the arrows, where his body's joints set, or sag, in a manner similar to the suspended chain. Our subject's joints are "set," resilient but not drooping.

Despite his body's structural arrangement our subject is neither stiff nor rigid. Rather his body retains a yielding quality, much like a sponge cake. His body's supporting joints, as well as his perineum (which serves as a floor for the abdominal cavity), are like water with the tensile continuity of its surface tension floating a needle. This is *sung*.

Forget Yourself

"Forget yourself," is advice I have often heard my teachers give in the past. Like many of the tidbits I have gleaned from them and fellow teachers (or students) along the way, I tend to extrapolate my own meaning from these gems. "Forget yourself," is advice pretty much intended to mean that we should practice our T'ai Chi without ego and learn to pay attention deep down inside to what is going on in our innermost selves with our bodies, our minds, and also the *Chi* energy flowing through our acupuncture meridians. This advice is all well and good, and we should all be so fortunate as to reach this pinnacle of selflessness through total self-awareness in our training. However, like many such dictums, the meaning can be applied variously and according to circumstances.

Right now, for example, I am thinking of interpreting the meaning of "forget yourself" quite literally. I am referring to those embarrassing and woeful moments when, suddenly, in the midst of doing your form along with others, you look around and realize that the whole rest of the class is practicing the wrong move, or so you wish!

Forgetting where one is in the form is quite common for novices and beginners who simply do not have their movement sequences hardwired into their bodies yet. For newer level students "forgetting" is just it what implies: *forgetting*. Newer students forget their form, yes, but not themselves. For more advanced practitioners, though, the surreal observation that your body is not at all where it is "supposed" to be may stem from causes other than simple memory failure. Certainly, any practitioner, regardless of skill level, can bring distracting baggage to his or her practice and fall out of step with the intended lesson at hand. But sometimes what happens is that you can just become so fully absorbed in the deeper aspects of your practice that your body zigs when everyone else's zags, and it is perfectly okay because you are still doing T'ai Chi. That is, until you realize your detour, and your bubble pops.

Though I have worked with many prominent and skilled T'ai Chi masters over the years, I have yet to encounter a master level teacher who is immune to this tendency. Even the best teachers incur occasional "memory lapses." No matter. By my way of thinking this simply serves as a reminder that even the most highly skilled teachers are, after all, human.

What to do when this happens to you? Well, obviously, you should "forget yourself." That is, let go of any ego attachment to the situation and just get back with the program. Holding on to dismay or self-judgment because you have missed a couple of moves only compounds any error. Once an error is manifest there is no undoing it, so chuckle, get over it, and move on to the next correct posture.

Quantitative vs. Qualitative

Students often enter into their T'ai Chi training with varied and wide ranging agendas. Regardless of how varied and wide ranging their agendas are, almost all students share two common goals, or expectations. First, students expect to learn a T'ai Chi form pattern as a central and supporting feature around which the rest of their T'ai Chi will be built. This is certainly a reasonable and realistic expectation given that the form aspects of T'ai Chi have been so widely disseminated in the media, and also because all T'ai Chi styles do, in fact, employ form routines. Secondly, most students expect that T'ai Chi will somehow enrich their lives as a result of their learning its form pattern. This, also, is a reasonable expectation, but one that is substantially more dependent on the student than it is inherent in the discipline.

Beyond having these general expectations, students may have little basis for anticipating just how these two distinct aspects of their agenda will weigh on each other as interdependent dynamics. Many students simply assume that learning the moves of the T'ai Chi form will, automatically and on its own, effect changes in their quality of life. I think this is a big leap, and one that may not necessarily play out quite as automatically as many students anticipate. Because students enter into T'ai Chi with a predictably superficial understanding of the relationship between form practice and its presumed impact on their quality of life they may find that their actual experience of T'ai Chi lands somewhere off the mark from their goals and expectations. This can become problematic for students, to a greater or lesser degree, during certain stages of their training. As their goals and expectations fail to materialize on schedule or in exactly the way they imagined, students may mistakenly take issue with their teachers, or even develop disillusionments about what T'ai Chi practice really has to offer them.

Students would be well advised to keep in mind that the quantitative aspects of their T'ai Chi and the qualitative experience of their practice are two separate issues. Ideally, these two issues will prove to be compatible and mutually supportive. But their interdependence is not inherent in the discipline and is likely to unfold only over time and in accordance with the student's diligence and intention. Learning a form pattern is a predictable and quantitative experience. The idea of learning the moves to a T'ai Chi form is usually pretty straight forward, even though the moves themselves, or the memorization of the moves may be challenging. Just how challenging this will be will likely vary from student to student. But the idea itself of gaining a skill, or knowledge about a skill, by sequentially assembling the pieces of material associated with that skill is, in all probability, fairly consistent with other learnings the average student has been involved with. Because the idea is most likely consistent with previous learnings, it is probably also the case that you have a pre-existing model for how the learning process unfolds. Simply put, T'ai Chi techniques and movement sequences are learned, sequenced, and accumulated one piece after another until you, eventually, learn the form routine in its entirety.

However, as I already noted, the T'ai Chi model does not guarantee a quality of experience commensurate with the acquisition of technical knowledge. Feeling yourself enriched by your learning experience is more subjective and qualitative than is the process of learning the movement patterns. The individual experience of T'ai Chi and its effects can vary from student to student or even for the same student from time to time. How you experience your T'ai Chi on any given occasion, or in general, in the perceived effect it has on your life will depend largely on your personal outlook, your mood, and certainly on the quality of your attention to and intention about your studies, not to mention whatever value you subjectively place on your T'ai Chi experience. Somehow, learning your T'ai Chi techniques quantitatively and experiencing them qualitatively must be interwoven, and closely so, in order for your T'ai Chi to become optimally valuable to you as an integrative experience.

The best way to accomplish this is to start by recognizing the difference between these two aspects—qualitative and quantitative. The quantitative aspects are the tools you have at your disposal. Though these tools may have a direct impact on your body's strength, flexibility, and relative health, only you can attach a qualitative value to those benefits. Your teacher can guide you and inspire you, your fellow students can support you, and your school or practice area can have an ambience conducive to T'ai Chi. But in the end you the student/practitioner are solely responsible for the manner in which you deem your experience of T'ai Chi to be of service and personal benefit.

Here are some tips to help you get the most, in terms of perceived benefit, out of your practice of the T'ai Chi form.

- Remember, you are not your form. If you find yourself struggling with some aspect of your form don't take it to heart. Of course, your form and your experience feel personal because they are yours. In trying times, it is best to step back and separate your ego from your practice. If you can do this, you will find yourself better able to enact corrective measures that work.

- Anytime your expectations for your T'ai Chi vary from the reality of your T'ai Chi, sit back and reassess your experience. It may be that your expectations are unreasonable. Or, it may just be that you need to make adjustments to the manner in which you train or perceive your T'ai Chi. By way of example, a student of mine underwent a serious personal health crisis, after which she was distraught that her T'ai Chi had failed to mitigate the circumstances or severity of her plight. Sympathy was in order at the time. But, at a later time, she and I spoke about how her expectations that T'ai Chi might somehow have rescued her from her situation were not reasonable.

- If you find yourself wallowing in uncertainty or despair, seek counsel in your teacher or fellow students. Often an objective perspective can offer clues or guidance that your emotional involvement in your own practice precludes.

- If there is some aspect of yourself or your T'ai Chi that you are dissatisfied with, find a quiet place to reflect and try to imagine yourself in a scenario more in keeping with your goals. Try to develop a sense of the gap between what you've already got and what you aspire to, as well as what is preventing you from bridging that gap. Once you have a clearer sense of any impediments you can try to adopt a T'ai Chi-like approach in dealing with those impediments.

- Keep in mind that the very masters of old who you may seek to emulate most likely incurred their own challenges and difficulties. Nobody gets to be good at T'ai Chi without undergoing some hardship. In Chinese, your ability to persevere in the face of hardship is called *chi ku* or "eating bitter." I say: "bitter now, better later."

Auxiliary Practice

Many people engage themselves in the study of T'ai Chi Ch'uan with the full hope and expectation that all their needs as a developing student will be adequately addressed by T'ai Chi form practice alone. This is a misnomer. Not only are there a range of T'ai Chi skills not adequately met by form practice alone, but practicing only the form is, at best, a slow boat on the road to proficiency.

Auxiliary training skills such as Pushing Hands, Chi Kung (Qigong), and piecemeal analysis of individual T'ai Chi techniques are necessary in order for you to develop a well-rounded grasp of T'ai Chi Ch'uan's many aspects. Unfortunately, because of the manner in which T'ai Chi is usually depicted in the various media, most folks arrive for their course of study with a unilateral preconception as to what T'ai Chi training entails, form practice and form practice alone. One of my students, who is himself a T'ai Chi teacher, shared with me how a newer member of his class literally threw up his hands in despair and stormed out of a group session. This incident, which caused everyone else in the room to look on in surprise, occurred whilst the teacher was guiding his class through some Chi Kung warmups. The disgruntled gentleman was heard to mutter on his way toward the door that the training exercises they were practicing looked nothing like the T'ai Chi form he had been trying to learn from his David Carradine home practice video.

Despite this fellow's sentiments to the contrary, I remain firm in my conviction that auxiliary training is a necessary complement to forms practice. I spend a good amount of time focusing on auxiliary training with all my students. In fact, that there are rare classes during which we never even get to practice the T'ai Chi form, so enamored am I with the value of examining and understanding all of T'ai Chi that is not *The Form*.

At times, this emphasis on auxiliary work can seem a bit tedious for newer students who may be hoping to add to their breadth of knowledge by tacking on the next move or two in their form sequence. My belief is that as eager as students may be to learn the next move, I am serving them better by broadening their resources and establishing a strong foundation in basic skills. Some teachers prefer to teach only the form first, and hold off on auxiliary methods until the student is further along on his or her path. As I have often stated, teaching methods vary widely, which does not necessarily make them more or less viable. No disrespect meant to other teaching methods, but my preferred approach is to give students a fuller disclosure of, and exposure to, the many possibilities that T'ai Chi holds for them right off from their earliest stages of training. Admittedly, this approach often means that students require more time to learn their form than if my approach were more straight forward and linear. But, it also means that students will possess a more encompassing grasp of T'ai Chi by the time they have completed their form through to the end.

Cross Associations

Every now and then, I reminisce back to that stage of my life when I had just come of legal age. As a young man, after eight years of hard style martial arts training, I wavered at the cusp of my adult life. I made a conscious decision at that time to get my house in order, having evolved beyond the indiscretions of my youth, by taking steps to plan more deliberately for my future and toward the realization of my personal vision. Simultaneously, I undertook the study of two separate disciplines.

The first of those undertakings was what proved to be my enduring pursuit of Chinese martial arts. This included my study of Kung Fu, T'ai Chi Ch'uan, Chi Kung, and other internal art studies.

The second discipline, which proved to be less pervasive in my life, but enduring nonetheless, was my study of therapeutic bodywork, or massage. Though I only indulged myself for a brief period of time at massage as a practicing professional, many of the lessons I learned from my experiences as a bodyworker remain with me still.

Nowadays, I find myself referencing those old lessons even as I continue to pursue my first passion in T'ai Chi Ch'uan. Specifically, what calls to mind my earlier experiences with massage are certain aspects of my T'ai Chi form practice. There seems to be a way that old memories of my earlier work, memories harbored deeply within my body, occasionally get prodded to the surface while I am engaged at form practice. What I find interesting is that for decades these memories apparently lay dormant. Only recently over the last 10 to 15 years, once I reached a certain level in my own practice, did these memories, and the knowledge latent in them, begin to percolate back to the surface with fresh insights.

These days, whenever I find myself deeply engaged in my practice of T'ai Chi, its rhythmic quality, the softness of touch, and the way I feel the contours of the air as my hands move through it all serve to evoke recollections of my earlier bodywork experiences (Figure 10-6). It is as if I can sense, all over again, what it once felt like to have another person's body beneath those hands, as my fingers searched knowingly for places that sought their counsel (Figure 10-7).

As the massage therapist I once was, I needed to perceive, and actively seek out, via my sense of touch, where exactly in whatever body I was working on its tension might be stored. Because tension in the body is often not merely held but actually *concealed,* I needed to pay attention for any nuances indicating resistance to my probing touch. Then, once found, pockets of tension needed to be dealt with in ways that facilitated disarmament and surrender rather than further entrenchment.

Now, decades later, these memories are all very evocative of qualities we regard as desirable in both T'ai Chi form practice and in the more interactive Push Hands aspects. The commonalities are compelling. A soft touch, a fluid rhythm, and sensitivity for the contours of energy and intention all lend merit to the practice of both deep tissue bodywork and T'ai Chi Ch'uan. My awareness of this leads me to

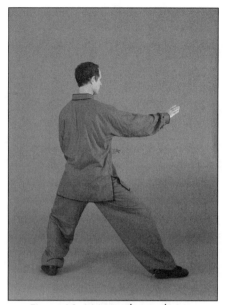

Figure 10-6 Notice the similarities
between the essential qualities
of this posture . . .

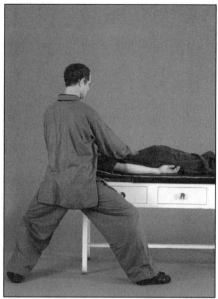

Figure 10-7 . . . and this.

conclude that therapeutic massage and T'ai Chi can be powerfully complimentary activities for those individuals who already practice one or the other.

If you happen to be a massage therapist, or even if you just practice massage recreationally, both your technique and the manner in which you administer it can be enhanced considerably by applying the principles of T'ai Chi posture and body structure while engaged in your work. For starters, this can help you to avoid strain and minimize fatigue while you work on others. Calling on your T'ai Chi skills can also help you to improve your actual technique by being better able to perceive what is going with the body beneath your hands.

If you are a T'ai Chi'er you might consider either learning some massage or just arranging to be on the receiving end of some good bodywork. I've already made a case for the benefits of practicing massage. But even just receiving deep tissue bodywork, aside from the obvious benefits of relinquishing limiting stress and tension, can help to reveal aspects of your own body (e.g., painful tension areas, muscular imbalances) that you might not already be familiar with. Bodywork can help you to know yourself, and knowing yourself is always an asset when it comes to T'ai Chi.

Mining Your T'ai Chi for Gold

One of my pet interests over the years has been the precious metals mining industry, specifically the gold sector. You might call it a romantic nostalgia for days of yore when prospectors combed the hillsides panning for their fortunes. Of course, today's industry is far removed from pack mules and gold pans. Still, from my perspective as a T'ai Chi teacher, I see some very interesting comparisons between the two endeavors. In both cases—mining for gold and learning T'ai Chi—success lies largely in one's ability to sift though impurities in order to end up with only the best stuff. This one similarity aside, there appears to be an inverse correlation between the process of mining ore for gold and the process of mining T'ai Chi for its own most precious qualities.

Over recent centuries, the gold mining industry has become more efficient with technological advances. In the old days, prior to modern extraction processes, refiners removed what gold they could from the ore that was mined, at least as far as was economically feasible, and cast aside the remaining ore, known as tailings. A blight on the environment, for sure, these tailings were not fully depleted of their gold content. As technological developments made the extraction process more efficient, the cost of refinement dropped accordingly. With new technology the old discarded tailings offered a ready and newly cost effective source of the Midas metal, even though the bulk of the gold had already been extracted. With additional technological advances even these old tailings may yet yield more gold, albeit less and less with each subsequent refinement.

In T'ai Chi we can also go back to mine and refine areas in our practice which have already been scoured over. Unlike the gold-laden ore mined from the earth, our T'ai Chi tailings become ever more profuse in the riches they yield.

When you first begin to learn T'ai Chi, you are limited in your ability to absorb its riches by your inexperience and by your lack of fluency at T'ai Chi's subtler essences. As you gain experience at T'ai Chi, instead of always moving forward to learn additional new material, you become better able to glean relevant and significant insights from aspects of your practice that you are already well familiar with. In T'ai Chi, the more time and effort you put into mining over your original lodes of learnings, the more you stand to gain by reviewing them yet again with further attention to their minutia and nuances.

Of course, if you merely repeat what you have learned in the past, without attempting to discriminate critically for nuances and deeper and more efficient connections in your body, you can hardly expect to make significant progress. Depth work requires depth attention and this, of course, is one of the reasons we practice T'ai Chi slowly. Also, body mechanics and connections aside, the same attention to perusal can be applied to how you experience the flow of Chi energy through your body. The secret in acquiring good T'ai Chi lies not in learning more and more in a linear sense, but in learning what you already know better and better. This is how you stand to gain 24-carat T'ai Chi.

Affecting the Mastery You Fancy

I recall how years ago when I aspired to certain T'ai Chi qualities that seemed beyond my grasp, I would role play those qualities in the privacy of my own practice. I would proceed through my practice imagining myself to be moving fluidly, or connecting my body, or issuing force as if I really had the ability to do so in the manner of some T'ai Chi master on high. No matter that I may have only been *affecting* those qualities, and perhaps poorly at that. The important thing was that I was "moving outside my box" and exploring new possibilities for myself. I was imagining the possible rather than the impossible. Now, years later, I realize just how beneficial that role playing actually was in helping me to grasp the qualities I yearned for.

At first glance, make believe and pretend seem more suited to young children than to reality based adult martial arts enthusiasts. Yet, can any of us honestly say that we have never envisioned ourselves as some highly skilled master while viewing a live or taped performance of T'ai Chi or Kung Fu masters in action. Of course we have all daydreamed at some point how it might feel to be every bit as skilled at T'ai Chi as we might hope one day to become. In truth, most of the realities we do actualize for ourselves as we move through life can be traced back to their inception as some small spark in our imagination. It would seem to make sense then that by indulging ourselves certain fantasies, we can increase the likelihood that they may, eventually, come to fruition.

I am reminded here of martial arts teacher and author Mark Salzman's description of himself in his book, *Lost in Place* in which he describes himself during his early teen years as an absurd young adolescent wearing skull caps and lighting incense in his cellar, all the while fancying himself as a Kung Fu monk. His account had me rollicking, both because it was hilarious, but also because I could relate. Mark subsequently went on as an adult to experience a measure of success and acclaim in Chinese martial arts prior to shifting his interests to other pursuits. My point here is that no matter how silly some behavior may seem at a time, it can still bode as a first step in the direction toward some real and significant accomplishment.

How might you make practical use of unconventional, even fantasy-based, behavior in your own practice? You can start by envisioning yourself as less limited by all the usual constraints in your life. The great majority of whatever constraints you live by are self imposed. Think about it. The only thing really standing in your way is you. If and when you are able to recognize this simple truth, you can then give yourself permission to behave outside those usual constraints.

We all put masks on in our lives and adjust our persona according to circumstances. The way you comport yourself around family or friends may well differ from the way you act in church, or from the way you behave in professional settings with your boss, co-workers, or clients. What I am suggesting here is that you try harnessing this ability in a deliberate manner to improve your T'ai Chi.

Imagine that you have an opportunity to apply for a leading role in a movie featuring T'ai Chi. Many actors who fill these roles are not nearly as skilled as their performance might suggest. Do you think David Carradine knew the first thing about being a Shaolin priest before he was cast for the role? Not likely. If you can imagine yourself as making your most convincing effort to try out for the role of some cinematic T'ai Chi master, you will have taken the first steps in extending yourself beyond your usual personal constraints.

Once you are prepared to try this, you can confine your focus to improving just one aspect of your T'ai Chi practice at a time. Naturally, in order to bring about improvement, you must be prepared to modify whatever aspect of your practice you decide to focus on (or else you won't be improving). You must be prepared to move beyond the usual constraints of how you comport yourself during training, including your perceptions about what actually comprises an effective practice session.

It will probably be easier for you to move completely unselfconsciously if no one else is around to witness your efforts. You must be able to envision yourself not as who you are now, but rather as whom you aspire to become.

Practice your form as you would imagine yourself practicing were you already a master of renown. Allow yourself to affect fluidity and gliding from your center, if fluidity and gliding from your center is what you need, or fa jin power release if that is what is on your agenda. Whatever qualities you aspire to, you can pretend as you practice what it would feel like and how you might perform if you already possessed those qualities. This is the gist of advice I impart to certain of my students when I feel they are stuck in a rut with intractable aspects of their training.

I would add that this imagining technique can work just as well for Push Hands as it can for the skills integral to T'ai Chi form practice. On more than one occasion, I have coached students whose characteristic stiffness appeared to preclude their ability to relax and move softly during pushing practice. When all other coaching advice seemed for naught, I would ask these students to move as they imagined they might move if they were already masters. I can't say this advice ever worked actual miracles. But it often did produce improvement, as students, in imagining themselves as masters, were able to affect uncharacteristic softness and fluidity, qualities previously beyond their grasp.

Of course, pretending, alone and by itself, hardly amounts to a comprehensive approach to gain mastery at T'ai Chi skills. But to the extent that role playing can help you move beyond your usual personal constraints to behave or perform in a manner more consistent with your ambitions, such practice can help bring the skills you seek more within your reach.

The T'ai Chi Learning Curve

One issue that pretty much escapes the attention of newer students, but which may warrant some attention over any extended study, is that of the learning curve. By this I do not mean wherever it may be that you fall on the T'ai Chi proficiency bell curve. Rather, I am thinking of another curve, one that gauges the breadth of your studies, versus the depth of your studies. This curve reflects *how much* you know, quantitatively, versus *how well* you know what you know, qualitatively.

Let us imagine that at one extreme representation of this curve are practitioners with a very narrow range of genuine expertise. Included in this group might be students who undertake their training with one teacher and stay with only that teacher, practicing and specializing perhaps in just a very narrow range of their teacher's overall knowledge. Over time these students can become specialists and quite skilled even to a point of being masterful at that one specific piece of T'ai Chi or internal arts knowledge. At the opposite extreme, we have those students whose approach is broader, so much so that their grasp of T'ai Chi remains superficial. In my experience, students such as these are actually quite a bit more common than those in the previous example. Students of breadth-not-depth are like collectors, and often take the approach of studying with many teachers, or even just learning from various media. Their approach is to acquire a wide and varied assortment of forms and/or weapon practices or internal skills, without really lingering to master any one piece of knowledge before continuing on to the next.

As is usually the case with curves, the great majority of folks fall somewhere amidst these two extremes. In my own case, I probably fell just a little more toward the collector end of the curve when I was young(er) and more ambitious. I accumulated an expanse of different material: Kung Fu and T'ai Chi forms and weaponry, Chi Kung practices, Taoist alchemy, and other internal arts disciplines. For example, I learned four different versions of the traditional 108-move Yang form from four different teachers. Yet, despite this, it was never my intention to simply collect for the sake of collecting. My sincere intention was to learn in the best way possible, and to attain the knowledge I sought through my own direct experience. However, because there was no way I could know in advance what answers some new learning might hold for me, I adopted the approach of learning many different things. Many of these learnings I ended up setting by the wayside, prior to settling myself down with a narrower focus. Even so, I found the experience of learning these many different teachings helpful to the extent that my experience allowed me to gain the very perspective necessary in order to effectively discriminate between which learnings were valuable enough to keep up and which ones warranted discard.

When someone learns a great deal about a small subject, as in the first example above, he or she can be said to have a *depth of knowledge*, albeit a narrow one (Figure 10-8). When someone knows a little bit about many different aspects of a more expansive subject, he or she has accomplished a *breadth of knowledge*, albeit a shallow one (Figure 10-9). I would argue that neither extreme represents an optimally encompassing approach to mastery. But that is not to say that you should exclude either approach in the overall scheme of learning and development. The relative value of either of these approaches can vary according to where you are at

Depth of Knowledge

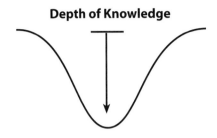

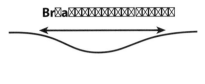

Figure 10-8 A narrow/deep learning curve . . .

Figure 10-9 . . . versus one that is shallow but wide.

in the grand scheme of your own training. As already noted in my own case, it was the process of accumulating knowledge earlier on in my studies that later afforded me both the opportunity to cull through my various learnings and the ability to do so.

Of course, in the long run a balance must be struck for best results. But as a general rule, the early years of study (especially for students who are younger) is a more appropriate time to experiment with and accumulate different practices for a breadth of knowledge. Then, as you grow older, with decades of practice under your belt, or even if you just embark on your studies at an older age, you will be in a position to determine which of these practices are most meaningful and beneficial for you, and you can narrow the focus of your attention to just those practices for real depth work.

What Might You Be a Champion of?

So what does it mean to be a champion? I began to contemplate this concept when a friend loaned me a DVD on T'ai Chi. This particular T'ai Chi instructional DVD declared on its cover, "The Champion Shows You How." Although the teacher in the video seemed to be skilled and knowledgeable, and had indeed been crowned as a fighting champion at a prestigious Asian competition, I was struck by the hollowness of his claim. Once a champion, always a champion? Yes, or no?

Not to belittle the achievement, but in most cases being a champion means only that one has outperformed others at some competitive endeavor. In other words, most champions only exist in relative comparison to others who have themselves failed to become champions. I speak from experience here, having been a "champion" myself many times over. In retrospect, each of those glorious occasions was only a moment in time, and hardly indicative of the more defining values I now hold for myself as a person. Being a champion may well imply admirable qualities such as tenacity, endurance, good judgment, or even just plain natural talent. But, as far as I can see, being a champion has very little to do with one's spiritual or emotional essence. Nor does being a champion, in the sense that champions are usually thought of, have anything to do with wisdom or tolerance or any of those issues such as heartfulness, peace and joy, intrapersonal growth, and self-actualization that I am fond of touting as part and parcel to one's evolving mastery of T'ai Chi Ch'uan.

I realize that there are perhaps a great many T'ai Chi practitioners who are highly skilled as a result of years or even decades of dedicated practice at T'ai Chi's more technical aspects, but who may have paid little heed to cultivation of the qualities and virtues cited above. In the cases of some practitioners, the practice of T'ai Chi may have inspired an appreciation and/or acquisition of these qualities and virtues as they endeavored along their paths. In other cases not. To all these hardworking individuals, who I hasten to add may be nothing short of fine people, regardless of how they may or may not have striven to achieve T'ai Chi's full personal development potential, I mean no disrespect.

> For me, and for many of those whom I teach, what brings T'ai Chi alive to actually improve our perceived quality of life, is the very way T'ai Chi can be employed to develop attributes such as heartfulness and personal congruence. All of T'ai Chi's more technical qualities are important, even vital, but so are its virtues. For by T'ai Chi's virtues, we not only become powerful as practitioners, we become more morally accountable as human beings and closer to becoming as at one with the Tao. Like *yin* and *yang*, technique and virtue must harmonize each other in order to offer the prospect of a more meaningful existence. Together, and in balance, these allow us to truly "live" our T'ai Chi.

As for being a champion and, I assume, a role model for others, this means only that one has once been triumphant. Fans and admirers may flock to champions because of their need to experience for themselves, vicariously, that winning feeling. This, of course, may only serve to reinforce a champion's belief in his or her own eminence. But it's all a facade. In the same way that fans admire their favorite champion in order to capture some of that winning feeling for themselves, a champion without his fans must, ultimately, look to his own counsel. In the end, it is much better to become your own "champion," a champion of yourself. Even though you may lack the resources, the opportunities, or the desire to prevail over others (a dubious accomplishment in any case), you can always become the best person to yourself and for yourself. And accomplishing your human potential, whether through your pursuit of T'ai Chi or by any other means, is a feat truly worthy of the accolades due any champion.

Simple Ordinary Learning or Transmission?

There is a very special kind of learning that is often referred to in the literature as occurring in the context of T'ai Chi. This particular sort of learning is not unique to T'ai Chi, but it is rare nonetheless, happening as it does under only under a narrow range of conditions. Furthermore, this particular kind of learning is not unequivocally available to all students. Yet there is no favoritism involved. That's just the way it is.

I am referring here to the kind of learning that occurs through *transmission* of knowledge. *Transmission* implies knowledge or understanding that has been passed down from one generation to the next. I mean by this knowledge that has been *attained* and understanding that has been *realized* in a very special manner as opposed to information that has merely been *conveyed* in an ordinary manner from one's teacher.

The student/teacher relationship is paramount in the pursuit of any martial art that espouses the development of character along with that of technique. Character development aside, the grosser mechanics of fighting technique or form patterns can easily be acquired by most anybody under casual circumstances. Even in the absence of a teacher, techniques and form patterns are the sort of information that may be obtained from books or videos. But the mentoring that traditionally accompanies the study of T'ai Chi or other martial arts allows for a much subtler and more essential transmission of knowledge from each generation to the next. This, of course, presumes a level of personal as well as professional development on the part of the teacher in areas other than technical martial know-how. The nature and the quality of transmitted knowledge will necessarily be linked to the teacher's knowledge of his art, but also to certain of his personal qualities, such as the way he or she practices respect, humility, and compassion. In order for transmission to occur, there needs to be a special rapport between student and teacher. This connection is not one of friendship, or loyalty, or well-defined roles, but of rapport on a less corporeal level. This kind of connection may exist even unbeknownst to either party (although, if so, this is more likely to be the case with the student), however cryptic that may seem.

My good friend, Jane Cicchetti has described a somewhat similar phenomenon that occurs in psychotherapy and in homeopathy and, I am sure, in certain spiritual traditions as well. In her book, *Dreams, Symbols & Homeopathy, Archetypal Dimensions in Healing* (Cicchetti 2003), Jane portrays this dynamic as part of a "healing alliance," whereby the patient and the health care provider are able to establish a special channel of communication. The essence of this dynamic is that clients often experience and voice their own process in alignment with the "language" and orientation of their therapist. Clients of behavioral therapists may both perceive and express their issues couched in behavioral terms. Clients of Jungian therapists more typically bring dreams to the table or make archetypal associations. Thus, the client and healthcare provider come to share a common language, so to speak, as per the particular healing modality of the provider. Once client and therapist have established this link, the therapy can unfold more freely and proceed less hindered by the usual obfuscations. In fact, establishing this special connection often facilitates insight on the part of both parties into the healing process.

Similarly, in T'ai Chi, the student and teacher must be correspondingly conversant with each other in order for transmission to occur. However, in contrast to the previously mentioned therapeutic modalities, this conversance, as it occurs in T'ai Chi, doesn't need to be expressed in so many words. It is often not based on verbal communication. In fact, a great deal may remain unspoken, for in T'ai Chi Ch'uan spoken words are but a secondary means of communication and not the language of choice. Regardless of whether a student's part in this rapport is expressed nonverbally or in some spoken fashion, the student must align with his teacher to a degree of fluency in the language of the body, or the language of subtle energies, or of warrior spirit in order to be truly receptive to whatever lesson is in the air.

Typically, those students who are very connected, or aligned, with the energies of their teachers make the most likely candidates for acquiring knowledge via transmission. The same lesson or lessons may be simultaneously within reach for all who are present, but certain lessons will only be accessible to students who are able to fine tune their learning antennae accordingly.

Before students can evolve to a ready state allowing for this kind of connection to occur, it is typical that many years of diligent study must be endured. Customarily, this is understood to mean many years with the same teacher. Over this span of study, the student may (reasonably) develop as one component of the student/teacher relationship some feeling of loyalty toward his or her teacher. And here I digress briefly, deeming a caveat to be in order. Loyalty is one quality this author feels is overrated as an ingredient in the pursuit of T'ai Chi excellence. Though not inherently bad, loyalty, when blind, extends beyond the bounds of responsible and appropriate respect and admiration. Blind loyalty is little more than a poor substitute for a healthy and well-developed sense of personal autonomy. It discourages true accountability to one's deeper self and may therefore taint any transmissions that are received. I encourage you to not make the mistake of confusing loyalty with true rapport in which the respect and admiration between student and teacher are mutual, and their connection genuine.

Transmission is not something that I, or other teachers, necessarily engage in by design, although we may on occasion attempt to orchestrate the necessary circumstances when we feel a student is well ready. Nor can transmission be measured or recognized or extracted from a curriculum like other kinds of learning. Yet it is there for all who are ready to receive it, and it happens when it happens.

Receptivity is the key, and the aforementioned "orchestrations" aside, it is up to the student to be receptive. A student's receptivity is not something that happens electively. A student cannot just decide and announce one day that he or she is ready for the subtler kind of learning that occurs via transmission. He or she must truly be ready, and this can only happen in its own time, regardless of the student's intent or awareness, or even his or her level of skill.

Even so, students can take steps to prepare themselves to be recipients of transmitted knowledge. In fact, such preparation is the essence of martial study. Diligent practice and perseverance over an extended course of study are what lay the groundwork in bringing the student into alignment with the teacher and the "frequency" of his or her transmissions. Students whose learning radar is attuned to just the movements of the body or the specifics of a technique will be limited in their abilities to absorb anything deeper than the lesson most superficially at hand. But students who, over time, are able to both cultivate their bodies and their character and develop that special sensitivity and rapport with their teachers may well find themselves the heirs to a special knowledge and, perhaps one day in a position to transmit that knowledge to their own next generation.

The Value of T'ai Chi Weapons Practice

Traditionally, weapons practice has been regarded as an important part of T'ai Chi training, at least for anyone who trains seriously and in a traditional manner. Yet, every now and then I encounter someone who is of a mind that weapons have no place in the scheme of T'ai Chi Ch'uan. Being a traditionalist, I am of a different mind. Naturally, I expect to meet the occasional skeptic whose lack of firsthand knowledge about T'ai Chi prejudices him or her against weapons. On rare occasions, I have even chanced upon otherwise knowledgeable internal arts teachers who dismissed weapons practice outright as being of no real value. Most often, though, I deal with novice level students who believe they want to learn T'ai Chi, but have little understanding of what the art is really all about. Their simple ignorance, for which they cannot be faulted, has them wondering what all these blades are for when they thought T'ai Chi was just about moving slowly and/or being at one with the universe. They didn't hear anything about swords and all from their home practice video, their T'ai Chi friends, or that article in the local paper. To them, swords, even slow moving swords, appear as sharp, pointy, scary looking things, the observation of which both fascinates them (a little) and intimidates them (a lot). So, what then does weapons training have to do with the practice of T'ai Chi Ch'uan?

First, let me acknowledge that there is a contemporary problem with how T'ai Chi weapons are perceived. The problem is that weapons are, well, weapons, and therefore perceived as such. In other words, the very idea of weapons is not PC (politically correct) in many circles. If you are already someone who practices with T'ai Chi weapons, then you probably don't give two hoots about the political correctness of weapons training. Nor should you, as long as you exercise reasonable common sense.

This brings to mind an incident that occurred some years back when one of my private students was returning home from class. He had just that day begun learning the saber form. On his way home he stopped to order a pizza, just like he did every week after class. As he waited in his car, with the door ajar, he sat fondling his saber, oblivious to the panic he was creating in hair salon next door to the pizza shop. Upon seeing this stranger with a sword lingering just outside their shop, the hairdressers bolted their door and called the police. Long story short: I ended up going to court to testify that my student was a bone fide martial artist and not some marauding psychopath. The judge gave my student his saber back, but not before issuing him a stern warning. Just a little common sense might have averted the whole fiasco. Even more so today than at the time this incident took place, the sociopolitical climate is not one that smiles favorably on weapons.

As a teacher of T'ai Chi (and of other Chinese martial arts that place a strong emphasis on training with swords, spears, sticks, and more), and as someone who has to deal with the public day in and day out, I do not have the luxury of appearing cavalier about weapons training. I deal regularly with parents whose Kung Fu youngsters want to learn sword forms ("they'll poke their eyes out," and "that looks so violent"). Plus, I have to be at all times sensitive to the way my school is perceived in the local community.

None of these issues required an inordinate amount of thought or attention prior to the terrorist concerns of 2001. Up until September, 2001, I had no problem waltzing into the airport and revealing that I had Kung Fu or T'ai Chi weapons in my possession, as checked baggage, of course. I rather enjoyed the curiosity that such disclosures elicited and the sometimes keen chatter about martial arts that often ensued. Times change. Nowadays I am more discreet when traveling with my swords, etc. In fact, I no longer check "weapons." Now I check martial art "tools," "props," "equipment," or "training paraphernalia."

Most dictionaries describe a *weapon* as some device designed to be used against another person for bodily harm. Of course, any casual object: hairbrushes, umbrellas, handbags, key chains, even newspapers, can be adapted in knowledgeable hands for fighting or self defense purposes. These items can be effective as weapons despite their design for other more benign purposes. From this we might construe that one's intent in *how* a device is used is as defining as the thought and intent behind its design in determining whether or not an item is, in fact, a weapon.

T'ai Chi Ch'uan makes use of several different kinds of weapons—straight swords (gims), and sabers (broadswords) being the most common (Figure 10-10). It goes without saying that such swords as these were originally intended and designed for use in actual combat and military scenarios. Their original design and purpose notwithstanding, the manner in which T'ai Chi swords are generally employed today is a far cry from the battlefields of ancient China. Sword practice, today, is clearly more in keeping with T'ai Chi as an artistic endeavor than with actual field combat.

When describing the use of T'ai Chi swords to new students or other interested persons, I emphasize their role as "training paraphernalia" rather than as weapons, per se. By my way of thinking this is not misleading. It is similar to the way that gymnasts practice floor routines but also use apparatus such as ropes, rings, and parallel bars. In order to continually challenge themselves, T'ai Chi practitioners can hone their skills by using such equipment as the straight sword, saber, or fan.

In any T'ai Chi course of study, it can be challenging, to say the least, to master your command of the four limbs you were born with. To add into this mix

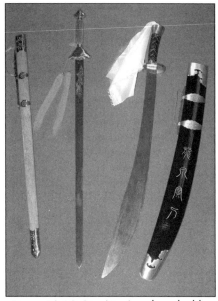

Figure 10-10 Gim (Jian), .a.k.a. double-edged sword, and Dao, a.k.a. saber or broadsword.

a sword or saber is just like adding on another appendage, a fifth limb. Of course, your T'ai Chi basic training remains paramount. The skill with which you wield a weapon can never exceed that of your T'ai Chi foundation practice. But the extra challenge of manipulating your weapon while maneuvering your body through intricate form routines can only enhance your sensitivity to where your arms and legs and torso are in relation to each other at any given moment.

In addition to the aforementioned benefits associated with T'ai Chi weapons training, there remains a hidden benefit. When students practice with weapons, especially if the practice is new to them, they may find themselves relapsing into old bad habits. Students who may have striven arduously in their regular form practice to resolve counterproductive habits such as raised shoulders or uneven postures may find themselves revisiting those same issues when wielding a sword. This observation lends credence to the idea that though a student may have apparently resolved certain undesirable issues, the tendency or susceptibility to respond unconstructively to unforeseen stressors may still remain. In order to be truly relaxed in T'ai Chi, it is not enough for you to merely relinquish existing stress and tension from your body/mind. Relinquishment alone, as valuable as it may be, is still of limited value if you remain subject to the tendency to retrench into old patterns when presented with new stressors. It is the tendency and the susceptibility to "stressing out" that you as a T'ai Chi'er must learn to evolve beyond. Therefore, weapons practice, by revealing any such residual tendencies, can create the opportunity for you to address them with corrective measures. Latent flaws in your technique are as undesirable as, and more insidious than, blatant flaws.

All said, T'ai Chi weapons can be a fun and relevant part of your practice. The unerring precision with which T'ai Chi weapons must be handled requires extraordinary focus and dexterity. Some practitioners are even of a mind that T'ai Chi swords are as antennae that can serve to influence or express your subtler energies. Regardless, there is little doubt that the challenge and demands of correct weapons practice can add considerably to your scope of knowledge, not to mention your enjoyment of any extended study of T'ai Chi Ch'uan.

Pregnancy, Low Back Pain, and T'ai Chi

This inclusion may seem a bit out of place, but it is a small token of my appreciation to all the pregnant women of the world, without whom (we should all bear in mind) there would be no T'ai Chi Ch'uan. This should also be of value to anyone, of either gender, who has lower back pain that is exacerbated by carrying excess weight.

I can't honestly claim I am inundated with pregnant T'ai Chi students, but every now and again a student becomes pregnant, or someone enrolls already pregnant. That, plus the clinical experience I gained years ago with my homeopathic practice, has afforded me some insight into the particular problems encountered by women during pregnancy. Unquestionably, the most widespread complaint I have encountered from pregnant women is that of low back pain in their third trimester.

I believe that T'ai Chi can be of great service in alleviating back pain as it occurs, or, even better, preventing back pain before it starts. T'ai Chi is based largely on body mechanics, which under normal conditions are fairly stable and predictable for any given individual over the short term. Pregnancy however, changes all that. A woman's body undergoes remarkable changes during the nine months she is pregnant, and for at least a short time afterward as well. Even though the expression of a pregnant woman's body mechanics may vary with her physical condition, an understanding of the underlying principles of body mechanics may provide some relief from the symptoms of lower back discomfort.

The amount of body weight that a woman puts on during pregnancy can vary widely. For the sake of example, let's suppose a woman puts on thirty to forty pounds, which is not at all out of the ordinary. If that additional weight were added over a nine month period and if it were distributed evenly throughout a woman's body it would still be an onerous burden, taxing her ankles, knees, and probably her lower back. The fact that a disproportionate amount of the weight added during pregnancy settles into the belly area adds tremendously to the challenge that a woman's body has in order to adapt accordingly. It is usually the failure of a woman's body to adapt optimally that results in low back pain.

I remember myself as a Boy Scout back in the '60s. I used to hike carrying a heavy load in a cheap haversack. The poorly distributed weight of that load gave me my first taste of low back pain. Six years later as a hippie hiking around the mountains of Colorado one of my few (and highly valued) material possessions was a more ergonomically designed backpack, which kept the weight of my pack high up on my shoulders, and my back free of pain.

The trick then, or so it would seem, when carrying extra weight is to distribute the weight you carry in the best manner possible. As regards pregnancy, the earlier a woman learns to arrange her body so as to distribute the weight she carries in the best manner possible the more time her joints, muscles, and connective tissues will have to adapt so as to minimize the effects of her burden.

A nonpregnant healthy woman practicing T'ai Chi ideally stands with a plumb centerline (Figures 10-11a and b). As a woman's pregnancy advances so does her belly. The usual consequence is that as the increasing size and weight of her child distends her belly forward, her lower back collapses inward as well, placing stress on the muscles, connective tissues, and bones and nerves of the lumbar and waist area (Figures 10-12a and b). If you were to notice this tendency in your own posture, your natural response might be to compensate by leaning your body forward to bring your upper body more in line over your lower body. However, this probably would not be much help. You'd still be out of alignment and now top heavy to the front (Figures 10-13a and b). This can easily be confirmed by having a partner push you gently from behind. Instead of being able to correctly redirect your partner's force down through your root, you will be unstable to the front (Figures 10-14a and b).

To correct this postural imbalance, and relieve the stress on your lower back, you need to extend your tailbone down and curl it under instead of leaning your body forward. If you only lean your upper body forward you do nothing to alleviate the bind in your lower back (Figure 10-15). Try extending your tailbone, first, down toward your heels, or heel (Figures 10-16a and b), and then curling your tailbone under (Figures 10-17a and b). This will stretch open your lumbar area and begin to release the tension that is causing your pain (Figure 10-18).

Leaning your body forward, as shown in Figures 10-13a and 10-13b, will fail to distribute your weight into your feet in a way that allows you to root down and keep good balance. Curling your tailbone under and forward, (Figures 10-16a and b and 10-17a and b), opens your *kua* and allows you to distribute your weight optimally between both of your feet from side to side, as well as lengthwise on each foot from front to back.

Even if you are close to full term and carrying twins, there's still no reason why T'ai Chi principles can't relieve or ease your lower back pain and allow you to keep a good root.

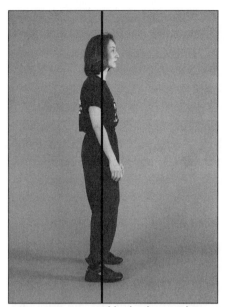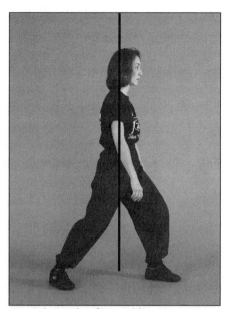

Figure 10-11a and b Plumb centerlines standing straight, and in forward leaning stance.

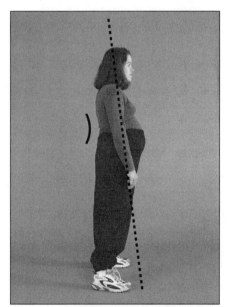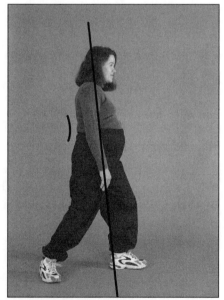

Figure 10-12a and b Exaggerated curvature of the lumbar spine.

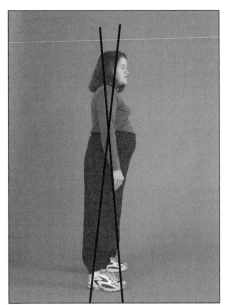 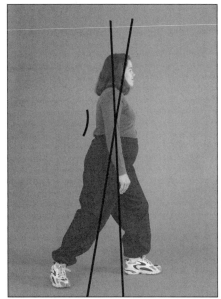

Figure 10-13a and b Leaning forward causes the person to be top heavy to the front.

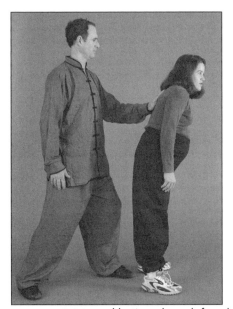 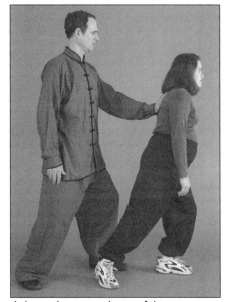

Figure 10-14a and b A gentle push from behind shows the unsteadiness of this position.

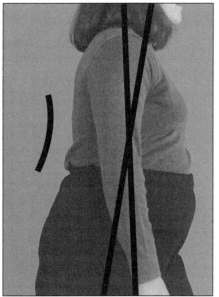

Figure 10-15 Close up. The lines show how the lower back remains bound when leaning the upper body forward.

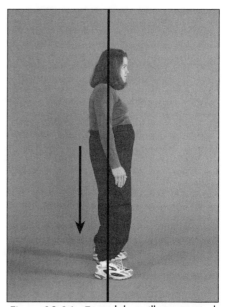

Figure 10-16a Extend the tailbone toward the heels if standing straight, or . . .

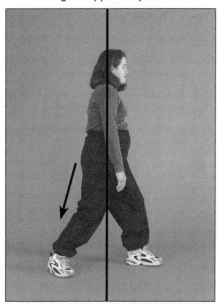

Figure 10-16b . . . toward the rear heel if in a forward leaning stance . . .

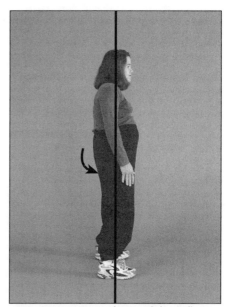

Figure 10-17a . . . then curl the tailbone forward like this, or . . .

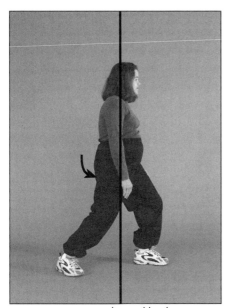
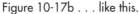

Figure 10-17b . . . like this.

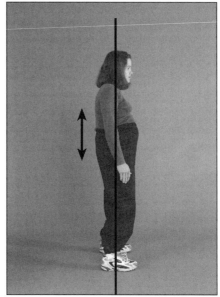

Figure 10-18 The lower back is now more open and expanded.

The Nature of Intention

Western science, including medicine and physics, has long concerned itself with cause and effect on the presumptive basis that all causes result in predictable effects, and that all effects stem predictably from causes. (One notable exception to this is the new branch of science based on chaos theory.) This premise lends itself well to the physical world where the components of cause and effect are generally identifiable and quantifiable.

However, not all of the 10,000 things lend themselves to scrutiny according to this western model, and particularly not those aspects of the human condition that are not exclusively indigenous to western culture. I speak here of *intention*, which, to the best of my knowledge, is a trait or characteristic common to all people wherever they may reside. Intention eludes scrutiny in any quantifiable sense according to the cause and effect model. In fact, intention seems to elude scrutiny from quite a few vantage points, even other than western science and medicine. This became all that much clearer to me as I vacillated in trying to determine if intention is best ascribed to the realm of trait, characteristic, ability, quality or, most probably, function. The inscrutability of intention does make it hard to classify, so much so that I'm anticipating a real challenge as I embark on my task of writing about intention. Nevertheless, I feel this is a necessary task, and I have the intention to do it.

In all martial arts, even including one as seemingly benign as T'ai Chi, intention plays an important role. Intention is regarded as especially indispensable with internal arts, such as Aikido, Hsing Yi (Xingyi), and T'ai Chi, in which it is used to regulate the self as well as to influence the manner and the effectiveness with which you deal with an adversary. Intention can make the difference between victory and defeat, and also between knowing oneself and wallowing in complacency. Beyond its value in interacting with others and keeping the ego in check, intention can effect all aspects of your T'ai Chi training and development. It can be a determining factor in everything from the frequency with which you commit to attend classes to the realization of whatever long term goals you set for yourself.

Let's start by taking a closer look at the semantics of intention in order to better grasp the concept. *Intention* seems roughly analogous to *conviction*, which implies a firmly held belief, but not necessarily action or behavior. Intention can also portend action, or the prospect of action, as if it were leading up to events about to unfold. Intention therefore seems to go beyond the implications of conviction and can become operative when a belief or an idea requires action that is deliberate.

Determination is another word closely akin to intention. Although, just as *conviction* failed confirm action, *determination* seems to me to suggest that action, as opposed to the mere prospect of action, is a forgone conclusion. Action that is forgone as a conclusion seems to extend beyond the domain of intention.

Purposefulness and *resolve* are probably the words most closely synonymous with *intention*. *Purposefulness* and *resolve*, like *intention*, denote a clear and undeviated sense of knowing what must be done. In my first book, I made reference to having witnessed and experienced first hand the ritual of fire walking. *Intention*, more so than any other factor, appeared to be the determining variable in whether or not someone was able to walk unscathed across a bed of hot coals. Believe me when I say you need a clear intention prior to taking that first step at a fire walk. To draw on a less extreme but still compelling example of applied intention, we have in my town a group called the Drowned Hogs. This group is comprised of several hundred people who take an annual plunge in frigid winter waters to raise money for charity. Most people eschew outdoor recreational swimming in the New England winter, and rightly so. But when members of this group set their minds with the clear *intention* of swimming at the designated date and time their bodies seem quite a bit more amenable to the activity than I would imagine any of them would be if one of their members were to, say, fall accidentally into the frigid waters. Intention, therefore, seems a likely precursor to notable accomplishments, great or small, or even unlikely, and certainly to those accomplishments that push the body or mind beyond its usual limits. Intention changes the odds in your favor when difficulty looms.

Even more so than whatever natural talent I may have been gifted with, or the excellent guidance I received from skilled teachers, it is my *intention* that I credit for advancing my Tai Chi to where it is today. I decided long ago that I had the intention to become a skilled T'ai Chi practitioner. Then, once I had realized that intention to a point that I had confidence in my skill level I developed another, related, intention, that of writing about T'ai Chi. Even more encompassingly, as I reflect over the last four decades, I realize that my life has been ushered into and through a series of actions and phases that were the result of deliberate, though not always conscious, intentions on my part. Some of these may at first glance appear to have been serendipitous or chance occurrences. But, I am sure even those were due to intentions I held that were already in place at some level. The part of me that has been most steadfast in seeing me through even my most difficult times has been my intention.

> **Though intention can be a conscious or an unconscious dynamic, it becomes most potent when the intention of your unconscious mind parallels exactly the intention of your conscious mind.**

Intention is a quality that might already be an important part of who you are, even prior to your gaining experience at T'ai Chi. As a pre-existing quality intention can help to enhance your acquisition of T'ai Chi's many features. The corollary is also true, that T'ai Chi and intention can be mutually enabling dynamics. T'ai Chi can enhance your personal clarity and your command of intention as a dynamic within your practice. Intention can help you to become rock solid steady and consistent, both as a T'ai Chi'er and as a person. Students often enroll with the idea in mind that T'ai Chi can help them gain some perspective, or a sense of control in an out-of-control life. As these students stick with their practice over time, T'ai Chi helps them to accomplish exactly that by integrating their different aspects and allowing them, even compelling them, to develop a clearer intention as to who they are, why they are, and who they intend to be. I would add that "rock solid steady and consistent" should not be confused with being rock solid inflexible. A powerful intention is not the same thing as a rigid intention.

Intention is something you can have about your practice. Intention is also a dynamic you can exercise within your practice. Acquiring or improving your own sense of intention can be as simple as taking the time (easy when you're practicing T'ai Chi) and attention to get focused on what you really want or need. Once you have a goal, task, or focal point in your sights, make the decision to assign it a priority such that your focus stays trained on that goal. Naturally, it helps if you keep your goals reasonable. The more you make a habit of practicing this, the easier it will become for you to establish a clear and reliable intention for yourself.

CHAPTER 11

Thoughts and Musings on Being a Teacher

One of the more defining characteristics of my first book, *Inside Tai Chi* (Loupos 2002) was the degree to which I volunteered self disclosure. I emphasized this particularly in the preface, where I offered a synopsis of my own studies with different teachers, and of the disillusionments that often accompanied those studies. Quite a number of readers, including several of those who reviewed my book in the press, commented favorably on that aspect of my writing style. When writing that first book, I felt it was important to give readers some sense of who I was and how I came to arrive to where I was in both my T'ai Chi training and in my life. I also felt it was only fair for me to self-disclose as I was asking a lot back from readers in return. I was asking them to take to heart what I had to share by trusting that they too could become reflective and self-exploratory about their own processes so that they likewise could grow to realize their full potential as the best T'ai Chi practitioners they could become. Though my request to readers was not framed overtly in so many words, it was actually an integral part of the underlying theme that defined that first book. I would like to offer something of a model for reflection and self-perusal in this chapter as well, for those of you who are teachers, and for those of you who have or are considering an ongoing relationship with a teacher.

It is very important to keep in mind that although T'ai Chi is an age-old discipline which is premised on certain principles and guidelines, the most important variable in anyone's course of study is not the objective aspects of the art, but subjective experience of the student.

> **T'ai Chi has no intrinsic value beyond the manner in which it serves to provide benefit to those who practice it. Of course, in order for T'ai Chi to profit its devotees it must be practiced correctly. Hence, the value of reliable guidance from teachers, books, or other media on how to go about learning in the correct manner. But, no matter what potential T'ai Chi may offer, we always come full circle back to an individual student's process and his subjective perception of how he learns and experiences his own T'ai Chi.**

To a very great extent the student's experience hinges on the relationship between student and teacher. For as long as I have been involved in martial arts I have heard discussions, opinions, and commentary about the teacher/student relationship. Mostly this stems from the perspective of the student's responsibility within that relationship. Conspicuous in its absence, to me at least, has been any significant comment on the teacher's responsibility to the student. It seems always to be assumed that the developing student's role and responsibilities must be hammered into the student, but that teachers are not held similarly accountable. Teachers, in all their wisdom, are presumed to know exactly what is right in all matters having to do with the student.

I question this wisdom. Every time I set out to conduct a class, I feel accountable to my students, not only to be the best teacher I can be but the best person I can be as well. Being the best teacher and being the best person means first and foremost being honest and genuine, hence my propensity for the aforementioned self-disclosure, even should that entail revealing some of my imperfections. In this chapter, I have decided to volunteer my thoughts on the topic of teacher accountability. I plan to include along with my own thoughts the pertinent thoughts of others, who I interviewed about this topic.

To Do or Not To Do

The teacher's first and sole responsibility is to guide the student in the best way possible to provide the student with an education in T'ai Chi Ch'uan. This statement is conspicuously open-ended in that it fails to spell out, specifically what "guiding" the student entails, or what "providing" for the student really means, or what exactly is meant by an "education in T'ai Chi Ch'uan." I would like to explore what all this means, but first I want to note that my open-ended statement was not as fully open-ended as it may at first appear.

There are certain details concerning the teacher's responsibility that were not mentioned, but which are, nonetheless, precluded by omission. For example, it is neither the teacher's responsibility nor his prerogative to use his power or authority to control, exploit, or disempower the student in any way. I have heard stories of teachers who have done just exactly this, either overtly and by design (criminal fraud, etc.) or, more often, inadvertently because of some aspect of arrested development on the part of the teacher. I know I am not a lone voice here as quite a number of the folks who responded to my survey questionnaire cited similar experiences. Examples of arrested development might include unresolved personality flaws, such as issues around anger, insecurity, impatience, avarice, or haughtiness, which can easily result in transferential or counter-transferential behaviors perpetrated against students.

I am not talking here about asking students to help out around the school with simple cleaning and maintenance, or the occasional favor that may occur between any two people who hold each other in mutual regard. I am not even talking about larger projects such as fund raising drives for one's school or freely offered volunteerism in regards to teaching duties or office help. I am talking about outright abuse of power. Flagrant financial exploitation aside, I have heard of teachers who derived personal gain by having students serve as unpaid laborers or craftsman on projects outside the school. I have known of students who were expected to cover up for, or even participate in, their teacher's substance abuse. And I have known of female students who were singled out for special treatment, despite their outright objections or lack of consensus in the matter, as playthings. Off the top of my head, I can think of five prominent martial arts teachers (thankfully only one of them a T'ai Chi teacher) within an hour's drive of me who, over the last two decades, have been arrested and prosecuted for crimes of a sexual nature perpetrated against their students. The worst case scenario is when children are involved. Exploitation of adults is bad enough, but abuse is particularly abhorrent when minors are involved.

I don't mean to scare readers off by blowing these concerns out of proportion. Criminal exploitation by martial arts teachers is hardly epidemic. It is the exception rather than the rule. Yet it is not unheard of.

> **Martial arts teachers, by my way of thinking, must hold themselves to a higher standard of behavior. We teachers have a mandate to serve as exemplars of right and righteous behavior for those we guide. However, when the standard of excellence we hold for ourselves exceeds the reality of our own psycho-emotional development, the stage is set for incongruent behavior as our shadow side seeks an outlet. Trying to behave as an exemplar is likely to prove nothing short of a facade if we don't pursue our own inner work.**

The truth is that most people live with some form or degree of arrested development. In the great majority of cases, this falls well short of blatant psychopathology. More frequently, arrested development issues are benign enough so as to be regarded as "adjustment" issues, if they even get regarded at all. To illustrate what I mean here's an example from my own life.

When I was a teenager I was strong willed and idealistic. Meanwhile, my father was strong willed and reality based with a limited tolerance for (my) idealism. The predictable consequence was that we clashed, and badly at times. I remember vowing as a teenager that if I ever had kids of my own I would never re-enact the same unjust and controlling methods toward them that were heaped upon me by my father. Well, lo and behold, it was twenty years later when I realized I was showing signs of repeating my father's pattern, a pattern of benign controlling issues that must have lain dormant all those years, with my own son. I was both horrified and bemused at the realization. Imagine me, the "evolved" teacher devolving in my own parenting methods. This wake-up call made me realize I had some work to do.

Consequently, I took the necessary steps to initiate changes in myself and in my parenting style. Now my son is grown, and we have a much easier and closer relationship than I ever had with my own dad.

I believe you can only be as good and effective a teacher as you are a person. At least I believe this is true for teachers of spiritual or personal development disciplines. So it is hard for me to imagine that the very same flaws, or places of "stuckness," that I recognized in my parenting style with my own son would not have been destined to have been expressed somehow in the way I taught my students had I not dealt with these issues when and as I did. I am sure the processing of my issues, as relatively benign for me as they were, contributed to my becoming a more balanced and effective teacher, and one less inclined to unconsciously heap aspects of my own shadow side on the students I guide.

Being a teacher of any martial art, and this includes T'ai Chi, can be an exhilarating and, to some, an inebriating experience. Martial arts, as a field, really is one of the last bastions of truly free enterprise in America. But this sword cuts both ways. In order to teach martial arts, one need not have achieved a degree in higher education, or even high school for that matter. In most states, martial arts remain an unregulated industry, meaning that anyone with enough moxie and even a rudimentary grasp of martial arts skills can open shop. For the most part martial arts are devoid of internal governing controls. Consumers who seek guidance in the martial arts often don't know the difference between T'ai Chi and Tae Bo. Consequently, novices are more or less dependent on their chosen teachers to educate them from the get-go, not only about a style's particular techniques, but also about its subtler features such as respect, etiquette, cultural aspects, compliance with the rules of the school, and with the teacher's presumed authority. Martial arts teachers are thus often imbued with what amounts to absolute authority once a student enters their doors. I do feel that this is probably a less pressing concern with T'ai Chi than with some of the more militaristic external styles. Even so, the upshot is that consumers (of any martial art) must beware to insure that they are really getting what they think they are paying for.

When a student and a teacher enter into a relationship, each party takes on a self-appointed obligation to meet certain agreed upon needs or wants of the other. In a student/teacher relationship, such as occurs in T'ai Chi, in which personal growth and development are part and parcel to the technical skills being taught, the teacher shoulders the greater share of the responsibility to insure that neither party deviates from its course. From the teacher's perspective a balance must be struck between the propensity of students to display transferential behavior and the teacher's own limits as a mere human being.

Because teachers shoulder the lion's share of responsibility in maintaining appropriate boundaries and behavior it behooves them to grow and evolve in all areas of their personal and professional development. This growth must extend beyond the technical and mechanical aspects of their martial arts, and also beyond their teaching skills and their business acumen, to include an awareness of what constitutes reasonable moral accountability to those they guide, provide for, and educate. As I alluded to earlier, all human beings have a shadow side. It is said that "power corrupts," and history has shown this to be true. Usually this statement is made in reference to military or world leaders or corporate executives. But this assertion can be just as true for individuals who wield power on a smaller scale in any case where they are disinclined to hold themselves accountable to both an inner moral authority and to the prevailing ethics and values of the society in which they live. Even T'ai Chi teachers must remain aware that their positions vest them with a certain power over others.

Teachers may, on occasion, appear as more or less aloof, or in charge, or laid back, or inscrutable. That is a teacher's prerogative. What is not okay is for teachers to be arbitrary with their students. By my way of thinking, arbitrariness transgresses the boundaries of accountability. Several examples of such capriciousness that I have witnessed or heard of come to mind. In one case a student arrived late for class and his teacher, out of the blue, punished him (an adult, mind out) by making him stand in the corner of the room. On another occasion a student was made to feel silly in front of his classmates for asking a question that the teacher wished to avoid answering. And in a third case, the teacher of another teacher made a unilateral decision to conscript his student's top student because he'd taken a liking to her. These are but a few of the examples I can cite off the top of my head. Just like any parent, there may be times when teachers, in their humanity, fail to measure up to the standards they or others set for themselves. At the very least, a teacher who oversteps the boundaries of propriety with a student needs to be able to recognize, or hear, that he has made an error and be able to say, "Oops, I'm sorry," or, "I was out of line."

In fact, it can be especially challenging for martial arts teachers, including those who teach T'ai Chi, to rein in their own power. The nature of our training is such that it increases our personal power and energy, and often in ways that we fail to recognize as such until well after the fact. In the absence of some internal means of checks and balances (i.e., conscious self-observation, meditation, counseling, or accountability through peer review), this increase in personal power can easily seek its own outlet, in the form of behavioral excesses or improprieties. Or, it can simply affix on to and exasperate pre-existing unresolved personal issues such as those mentioned earlier. You need only imagine someone with unresolved anger issues or poor self-esteem with martial power added into the mix going on to become a teacher. Augmenting unhealthy anger, or compensating for rather than actually mending low self-esteem, are examples of how martial power, even in a teacher, can aggravate one's shadow side.

The teacher's greatest responsibility therefore must be to himself, and only by extension to the student. The teacher must grow for the teacher first. Only when a teacher has harnessed his own ego (or at least engaged himself in that process) can he be truly available as an honest and congruent inspiration to those he guides. Anything less is a misrepresentation of the best that T'ai Chi has to offer.

Guiding, Providing for, and Educating Students

Guiding, providing for, and educating students in their quest for proficiency at T'ai Chi are closely interwoven. All students need guidance. That T'ai Chi amounts to unknown territory for students who are new to their studies is a given. Of course, new students with previous experience at T'ai Chi, or anyone who is shifting sideways into T'ai Chi from a background in some other internal discipline such as Bagua or Hsing Yi, may prove an exception to this rule. Short of this, the likelihood is that the full scope and nature of T'ai Chi Ch'uan will be as alien as some foreign language to the T'ai Chi novice. Therefore, it is the teacher's responsibility to guide his charges in navigating their new territory. Quite a lot of what is entailed in that navigational process from the student's point of view was covered in detail in my second book (Loupos 2003, chapter 1).

The teacher's role in the guiding process entails being sensitive to the student's preferred learning modality and learning abilities. In other words, the teacher needs to figure out how the student learns best. A teacher cannot expect good results from showing a student something that the student is incapable of seeing. Nor should a student be expected to learn at a pace set arbitrarily by the teacher without due regard for the student's ability. Usually, a teacher can ascertain how students learn best by asking them if they have any special learning considerations (examples of which might include dyslexia, stroke, loss of hearing, or balance issues), and by observing them during their initial attempts at learning. How individually any given instructor can cater to the specific needs of different students will vary according to the circumstances. Private instruction offers plenty of opportunity for "personalized" attention. Larger group classes may be less conducive to one-on-one attention, and martial arts camps even less so. Regardless, the teacher should make a reasonable effort to remain sensitive at the least, even if less than fully responsive, to each student in his or her class. One exception to this level of regard might be accelerated learning venues, such as camps or seminar intensives, at which (possibly many previously unknown) participants are informed prior to signing up what level of training is to be expected.

Of course, teachers cannot be expected to magically know what students fail to reveal about themselves. If a student is aware that he or she has some special learning consideration, such as a learning disability or a physical limitation, it is that student's responsibility to bring the teacher up to speed. By way of example, I have one long-time student who is quite intelligent and reasonably well-coordinated. But she has a minor learning quirk in that she processes information best at a slightly slower pace than I generally present it. Knowing this as I do (after she revealed it to me a full year into her training), has allowed me to be more sensitive to her needs. I often try to repeat instructions for her, using a different choice of words, in order to give her processing methodology time to catch up. Or, I may simply be more patient if she fails to get some lesson or guidance the first time around. In this woman's case, her critical analysis as she goes along is part of how she processes information. Her situation actually amounts to a perk for the rest of the class in that her critical thinking occasions some very sharp questions, my answers to which enables the whole class to benefit. In short, this means that the teacher must be sufficiently skilled that he or she can adjust the teaching methods according to how a student is best able to learn. In an informal survey that I conducted recently, respondents were more or less unanimous in their opinions that teachers should be very sensitive to their needs during instruction time.

In my classes, I periodically ask students how they feel their training is proceeding, if their expectations are being met, and how that might or might not be the case. I feel that though it is my responsibility to have an overall plan for how students' training unfolds over time, it is also my responsibility to try to engage students as conscious participants, co-conspirators if you will, in that plan. Naturally, not all students are the same, and there are wide variations in the assessments that students have of themselves, their progress, and their potential.

A Survey

In the section that follows, I have compiled submissions from T'ai Chi teaching colleagues and students that give some voice as to how others perceive the role and responsibility of teacher to student. I sent out a questionnaire to a small sampling of several dozen T'ai Chi'ers in which I asked practitioners to share their thoughts on the accountability of teachers to students. I included some teachers in this survey because every teacher has been a student.

Some of what respondents had to share was interesting but predictable in terms of what is thought to be reasonable accountability from teachers. For example, when asked, "How much personal disclosure a teacher needed to volunteer to his students?," the majority of respondents stated that they felt any personal disclosure beyond anecdotes to illustrate points being made in class was unnecessary. Other questions elicited responses that were less predictable and more diverse.

Aside from all the serious responses I received, one student, who fancied himself a comedian, tendered a response that was thoroughly facetious. Submitted in jest, it ostensibly offered nothing of redeeming value to my survey, and hardly warranted inclusion here. But as I chuckled over his response, I began thinking, in all seriousness, that sometimes what students have going on in the depths of their psyches can represent quite a departure from what we teachers might *imagine* is going on, the upshot being that teachers need to be wary of stereotyping their students. This association also served as a reminder that the lessons we choose to learn both from T'ai Chi and about human nature can be closely interwoven and may be culled from the most unlikely places.

Just as compelling, though, as "what" people wrote was the reminder that students have, and are willing to voice, their expectations and their hopes, as well as what they want and think they deserve from their teachers. If you are a teacher reading this, you might want to think back to when was the last time you asked your students what they expected of you!

Here now are the results of my survey.

I asked about, the level or nature of personal disclosure that respondents felt teachers should ask of students. As I anticipated for this question, responses ran the gamut from "none" to "teachers should ask about any physical or emotional disability" to "enough to be able to support students in their learning when they become stuck" to "leave it to the discretion of the student." One respondent related how her teacher had asked students to self-disclose during a Push Hands session, and how the information that was volunteered by her partner helped her to become more aware and filter out preconceptions she had about her "opponent." The most noteworthy opinion on disclosure came from a young T'ai Chi student who had just recently begun teaching his art. "A student teacher relationship needs some sort of disclosure, simply because it is a relationship. Regardless of the willingness of either party to disclose there is going to be some form of disclosure, whether it be verbal or by gesture. One needs to remember that sometimes even not saying something is saying something."

When asked, "How sensitive a teacher should be of the student's energy and space when attending class?," respondents uniformly felt the teacher should be held to a very high standard: "extremely sensitive," "in tune with my energy," "that is the teachers job," "very sensitive, because people's attitudes, energies and relative comfort zones change." One lone voice said he, "expects nothing when training with my teacher" and felt it was his job to "subordinate my energy and space to the energy and space of what I am supposed to be learning." It would seem here then that most students expect quite a lot from their teachers in terms of teachers "sensing" where the students' energy is at in any given class.

None of the respondents reported having a marked preference for following along silently while their teacher guided, versus receiving verbal guidance while practicing the form. Most said they preferred some variation on a combined approach. One respondent did add that, "being silent is a powerful part of the learning." All said they found it helpful when a teacher repositioned himself during form practice to provide all students with good vantage points. Several respondents added that they found it helpful when teachers designated advanced students or assistant instructors to strategic locations for less experienced students to follow along.

Respondents expressed strong opinions on the subject of teachers offering public corrections during group class. All agreed that public corrections were to be expected as part of one's studies, some even to the extent that learning to accept criticism was an important part of T'ai Chi training. Most respondents stipulated, however, that corrections should never take the form of putting the student down in any derisive manner: "corrections in public can spawn multiple conversations on structure, technique, etc.," "make corrections, but not at the expense of the student." Almost uniformly, respondents registered their opinions that teachers should be strict, but not tyrannical, in requiring behavioral compliance from students during class. This same sentiment was echoed broadly in regards to the standard of excellence that teachers should expect from their students. One person wrote that teachers should "be strict in requiring compliance, otherwise you'll have ten people all claiming to do the same thing yet look totally different. At some point you won't recognize your own art/style." As this comment was submitted by a fellow teacher, it wasn't surprising that his main focus took into consideration the long-term best interests of his art. One woman suggested that if teachers were too demanding then "some folks will find the lessons burdensome, especially women who may feel that everything/one else in their lives is demanding."

When asked if they felt free to express needs, wants, or desires to their teachers, I was surprised at the degree to which respondents expressed deference on the matter. "No, but this is mostly my own fault for not taking responsibility for my own learning process." Another person offered that it seems "disrespectful to impose on your teacher." Other respondents wrote "Let them [the teachers] decide what is best for your training"; "[students] must fall into the curricular of the teachers' teaching"; and, "[teachers are] not there to get involved in therapy or the expression of needs, wants, and desires." These comments typify the responses submitted for this question. Speaking for myself, I would have preferred to see responses to this question evidence more empowerment and initiative on the part of students in expressing their needs. Students who fail to express their needs, as a first step in negotiating how those needs might be met, can hardly expect to count on their teacher's omniscience in all matters having to do with their studies.

I asked if and how teachers should offer praise to students. Across the board, respondents were in favor of praise as a means of recognizing students' accomplishments and motivating them in their studies. The only caveat was that praise not be used to show favoritism. In an interesting twist, one respondent advocated "words of encouragement" rather than outright praise, insisting that, "too much praise can spoil the student."

The issue of respect between student and teacher elicited more varied opinions. Everybody seemed to be in agreement that mutual respect was important. However, there was some divergence as to how that respect should be best expressed. One respondent felt that teachers were showing respect for their students simply by virtue of sharing their art. More widely embraced was the opinion that teachers must earn the respect of their students, but also that teachers are responsible for creating the energy of respect in their teaching environments.

Another of the questions I asked was what responsibility teachers had to their students in the case of diverging agendas, such as when students and teachers have differing opinions about how a student's training should progress or evolve. I have to admit to being taken somewhat aback by the responses I received. There was almost a line drawn between the responses I received from teaching colleagues and those I received from students. The comments I got from students could be pretty much summed up by the following comment: "[The] teacher should recognize each student's goals and respect them." This is hardly unreasonable by my way of thinking. One student did volunteer her opinion that "the teacher is in charge and the teacher need not recreate his/her agenda for the student."

The teachers who responded displayed a surprisingly hard line in answering this question. Several teachers suggested some variation on dismissing the student, although one did suggest softening the blow with a refund on the way out the door. One teacher even went so far as to say, "it's my way or it's the highway." Teaching respondents were similarly rigid in their opinions on how to deal with "difficult" students. Only one teacher respondent opined that, "If [my own teacher is] not ready to teach me something, then I have to respect that." He went on to qualify his statement by adding that if the teacher's "knowledge is dangled like a carrot, then I'm gone."

In answer to the question, "Should teachers *just* teach T'ai Chi technically, or should instruction include; guidance, philosophy, history, personal anecdotes?," all respondents advocated the inclusion of nontechnical features as essential to the learning process.

I wanted to know how demanding both teachers and students thought teachers ought to be of their students. Though a number of respondents elected not to answer this question, those who did were pretty gung ho in their consensus that students, "must come prepared to learn," and that, "teachers should push their students to their limits, or even beyond." Frankly, I'm not swayed by the majority opinion on this one. I personally like to work hard. But I also have had quite a few students who fall short of this mentality. Perhaps if I'd phrased my question a little differently, more of the quieter types would have spoken up. One respondent did stipulate that a "teacher should never expect a student to do anything that he himself can't do." Again, I'm a dissenter here. Double standards aside, I think that it is perfectly reasonable for teachers, especially for those who may be older (as I hope to be someday), to expect their students to surpass them in their abilities and their skill levels. I can think of no greater accomplishment than helping students to evolve to a level of expertise that is equal to or beyond my own. The only way to accomplish this is by raising the bar high.

Another, apparently provocative, question addressed the issue of teachers socializing with their students outside of class. I was surprised that so few respondents indicated their approval of extracurricular socializing given that I know so many teaching colleagues who do socialize with their students, with no apparent ill effect. Most respondents nixed teacher/student socializing, especially with the opposite sex. Students who were the same sex as their teacher tended to be more casual on the matter, "I see no reason why T'ai Chi instructors should not socialize with their students. I consider my own teacher my friend and have often participated in social events with her." Based on the responses I received, I'm surmising that teacher/student fraternization outside of class is frowned upon more as a matter of policy than as a practical matter.

Respondents were even more emphatic in expressing their intolerance of more blatant forms of inappropriate behavior. The litany of unacceptable indiscretions perpetrated by teachers against students included "loosing their temper, putting a student down, cheating, dishonesty, bringing their personal problems into the class, borrowing money from or lending money to a student, entering into business deals with students, asking students to recruit for them too much, and forcing a student to choose allegiances," as well as, "not touching teenage girls who may jump to erroneous conclusions about being touched and then develop a crush on the teacher." Whew!

Happily, this foregoing list did not seem to preclude teachers expecting their students to contribute back to the school in various ways. Most respondents felt is was okay for teachers to expect a little volunteerism around the school, such as helping out with less advanced students, helping to keep the school clean, and being available to help out for special events and projects. "Students should be willing to give back to their school or teacher. Volunteering for events to promote the school and assisting with less advanced students is really all part of the learning process."

Of all the responses I received, the most poignant of all was submitted in by a student who chose to sum up her thoughts in a single paragraph rather than answer each question in turn. Her submission has been paraphrased here:

Martial arts teachers need to be responsible for their own inner work, meaning their mental and spiritual health, as well as their outer work. The biggest challenge in the martial arts is dealing with one's own shadow side. The outer enemy is but a pittance compared to one's own darker forces. Martial arts teachers who ignore this inner work may inadvertently seek balance in less healthy ways, such as addictive behaviors involving alcohol, sex, or power. In this regard martial arts teachers may not be all that different from most other people. Yet there is a difference. With the increase in energy that accompanies the practice of martial arts, and because teachers often have many students looking up to them, teachers may feel less accountability and have a greater propensity to overstep appropriate boundaries with students. If martial artists, and especially martial arts teachers, included more of this inner work in their practice and truly understood its value, they would make a great contribution to the training of others. Outer work, of course, is important. But it is this inner training that creates the true spiritual warrior.

In Summation

In the end, a rewarding teacher/student relationship depends as much on what the student wants and needs from the teacher as it does on what the teacher brings to the table. In order for any relationship to be optimally rewarding both parties must be clear and unambiguous about their roles and their contributions; otherwise, the relationship is dysfunctional and ill-fated. Of course, like any other relationship, one that occurs between student and teacher may have its high points and its low points as it evolves over time. This is natural and to be expected. On the whole, though, a healthy relationship must be founded in mutual respect and regard as much as in a desire that the needs of both parties be adequately met.

It may well be that you are perfectly okay with a teacher who shows you how to practice T'ai Chi Ch'uan and nothing more—that your teacher be someone who merely guides you through the moves of a T'ai Chi form pattern until such a point as you are able to practice on your own. If there is the added fun of practicing along with others whose company you enjoy, so much the better. Taken to a deeper level, you may prefer a teacher who inspires you—someone who is able to help you see that T'ai Chi can be useful beyond its most superficial expression as a body discipline or as a means of relaxing and reducing the effects of stress. Or, if you are fortunate, and so inclined, your teacher may become someone who touches your soul, and who helps you to grow and experience your T'ai Chi as a living philosophy. In such a case your teacher may become a mentor, a colleague, and even a friend.

References

Bennett, Bradford C. *Somatics Magazine Journal of the Mind Body Arts and Sciences,* "Tai Chi, A Somatic Movement Art." (Available for reading at somatics.org. Go to http://somatics.org/somaticscenter/library/bbc-taichisomatic.html.).

Cicchetti, Jane. 2003. *Dreams, Symbols, & Homeopathy, Archetypal Dimensions of Healing.* Berkeley CA: North Atlantic Books.

Davis, Barbara. 2004 *The Taijiquan Classics.* Berkeley CA: North Atlantic Books.

Hanna, Thomas. 1988 *Somatics: Reawakening the Mind's Control of Movement, Flexibility, and Health.* Harper Collins.

Loupos, John. 2002. *Inside Tai Chi: Hints, Tips, Training Process for Teachers and Students.* Boston: YMAA Publication Center.

Loupos, John. 2003. *Exploring Tai Chi: Contemporary Views on an Ancient Art.* Boston: YMAA Publication Center.

Newton, Isaac. 1687. *Mathematical Principles of Natural Philosophy.*

Salzman, Mark. 1996. *Lost in Place: Growing Up Absurd in Suburbia.* Vintage Books.

Resources

Taijiquan Journal. 612-822-5760. info@taijiquanjournal.com.
Tai Chi Magazine. Wayfarer Publications. 800-888-9119.
Journal of Asian Martial Arts. Via Media Publishing Company. 800-247-6553.

Glossary

10,000 Things

Lao Tsu's (Lao Tse) reference in his classic *Tao Te Ching* to all things under Heaven that ever were, are, or shall be.

Bagua (Pa kua)

One of China's Three Internal Treasures, Bagua is an umbrella term encompassing any one of eight different animal systems, all of which are characterized by twisting and coiling movement patterns or techniques and premised on the eight energies stipulated in the *Yi Jing: The Book of Changes*.

Body/Mind

I believe the term body/mind accurately reflects the integrative approach of T'ai Chi at its best. In truth, the body, except possibly under rare and extreme medical circumstances, never exists in absence of the mind. Nor does the mind, except perhaps in rare esoteric circumstances, exist separate from the body. I have never been able to delineate satisfactorily between the two.

Bubbling Well (*Yongquan*, K-1)

This first point on the Kidney meridian, at the bottom of each foot, is useful for rooting physically and energetically in T'ai Chi. You may locate this point by scrunching your bare foot and finding the center of the crease just behind the ball of the foot.

Chi (Qi)

Most simply and accurately described as life force energy. For the purposes of this book, one may regard Chi as that energy that animates us as living beings.

Chi Kung (Qigong)

This is a term used to describe practices that combine the attention and intention of the mind with a conscious and deliberate attention to breath and/or movement. Use of this term is generally confined to a rather wide range of exercises adjunct to Chinese Kung Fu, T'ai Chi, or other internal art forms. Different Chi Kung practices can be categorized as simple, formulaic, or medical.

Dantian (CV-8)

The body's physical and energetic center, the Dantian can be experienced just behind and below the navel. It is a place where we receive nourishment and Chi pre-natally and remains a place where Chi can be safely stored and cultivated throughout our lives. (This, actually is just one of three *dantians*, the other two being located at the Heart Center and the Third Eye.)

Dao (Tao)

Universe, Heaven, all that was, is, and shall be. What came to be after there was nothing. The Dao is understood to be a self-regulating harmonic force.

Ego

The conscious, rational component of the psyche.

Fa Jin

Term used to describe the execution of a move in T'ai Chi that is explosive and spirited and augmented by a release of Chi energy.

Five Thieves

The five senses: hearing, sight, taste, feeling, smell.

Feng Shui

Literally, wind and water. Feng shui is an ancient form of divination designed to optimize the harmony of one's environment.

Homeopathy

Homeopathy is a nontraditional medical system, rooted in 17th century Germany, and promulgated on the theory of likes being used to cure likes, versus the concept of "anti's" so prominent in traditional western allopathic medicine.

Hsing Yi

(Xingyi) One of China's Three Internal Treasures, Hsing Yi is known for it powerful and explosive techniques. Hsing Yi is also known as *mind boxing* due to the prominent role of intention in augmenting its martial techniques.

Li

Force which is founded in strength and muscular effort, and therefore regarded as external in nature.

Lordosis

Abnormal forward curvature of the lumbar spine.

***kua* (Qua)**

The *kua* is a general term used to identify the loin/groin area, but may be specifically understood as a reference to the inguinal crease that runs externally from approximately the forward crest of the ileum downward and inward to the pubic bone.

Miasm

In homeopathy miasms are generally regarded as inherited (although sometimes acquired) predispositions to disease.

Proprioceptors

Sensory nerve endings located in soft tissue and elsewhere in the body that serve to provide a sense of body position for balance.

Parasympathetic nervous system

Component of the autonomic nervous system that controls the body's relaxation response.

Push Hands

Interactive aspect of T'ai Chi practice wherein two individuals engage in cooperative or competitive sensitivity drills, either prearranged or spontaneous.

Shadow side

According to C. G. Jung, one's shadow side is the darker and unacknowledged aspect of one's personality, roughly the equivalent of Freud's id, or pleasure seeking self.

Sung

A particular quality of relaxation which, in the context of T'ai Chi, strikes a balance between total softness and tensile continuity.

Sympathetic nervous system

Component of the autonomic nervous system that controls the "fight or flight" mechanism.

***Ting Jin* (Listening skill)**

Ting Jin denotes one's ability to listen, or more accurately perceive, through the sense of touch, where an opponent's energy is, or even what his intentions may be, simultaneous, or even prior, to their being manifested as an action. To avoid confusing internal arts neophytes and keep things simple, I've opted to employ this one term broadly as an umbrella concept to encompass a range of related intrinsic T'ai Chi qualities including Tung Jin (interpreting skill), Tsou Jin (receiving skill), Hua Jin (neutralizing skill), and Yin Jin (enticing skill), among others.

Wu Chi

In Daoist cosmology, Wu Chi was the state of nothingness, or void, before there was anything.

Yin and Yang

These two forces represent polar opposites and exist as relative and necessary complements. Yin is regarded as feminine, dark, receiving, yielding, etc. Yang is masculine, light, issuing, solid, etc.. Neither is absolute, and either in extreme ultimately begets its opposite.

About the Author

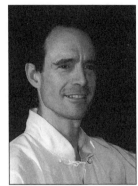

Sifu John Loupos, founder of the Jade Forest Kung Fu/Tai Chi school, has taught martial arts since the age of fifteen. His studies include Okinawan Karate along with several Chinese Kung Fu systems including Bak Sil Lum, Choy Lay Fut, and Praying Mantis, plus Yang style T'ai Chi Ch'uan, Liu He Ba Fa, Hsing I, and Bagua. John also practices and teaches Chi Kung and energy oriented meditation disciplines. He holds a B.S. in Psychology, has a background in Classical Homeopathy, and is currently pursuing studies in Hanna Somatics.

John specializes in T'ai Chi Ch'uan as an inter- and intra-personal communication modality and enjoys traveling to conduct seminars for educational and corporate entities as well as for other schools. He currently lives at the shore in Hull, Massachusetts, and busies himself with writing and teaching at his main school, Jade Forest Kung Fu/T'ai Chi/Internal Arts in Cohasset.

The author welcomes comments and questions from readers. Please submit correspondence to the Jade Forest Kung Fu/Tai Chi Web site, www.jfkungfu.com, or e-mail directly to jadeforest@comcast.net. Correspondence may also be submitted in care of YMAA Publication Center.

Index

COMPLETE BOOKS FROM YMAA

COMPLETE VIDEOTAPES FROM YMAA

more products available from...

YMAA Publication Center, Inc. 楊氏東方文化出版中心

4354 Washington Street Roslindale, MA 02131
1-800-669-8892 • ymaa@aol.com • www.ymaa.com

COMPLETE VIDEOTAPES FROM YMAA (CONTINUED)

CHIN NA IN DEPTH—COURSE 4	T039/035
CHIN NA IN DEPTH—COURSE 5	T040/124
CHIN NA IN DEPTH—COURSE 6	T041/132
CHIN NA IN DEPTH—COURSE 7	T044/965
CHIN NA IN DEPTH—COURSE 8	T045/973
CHIN NA IN DEPTH—COURSE 9	T047/548
CHIN NA IN DEPTH—COURSE 10	T048/556
CHIN NA IN DEPTH—COURSE 11	T051/564
CHIN NA IN DEPTH—COURSE 12	T052/572
CHINESE QIGONG MASSAGE—SELF	T008/327
CHINESE QIGONG MASSAGE—PARTNER	T009/335
COMP. APPLICATIONS OF SHAOLIN CHIN NA 1	T012/386
COMP. APPLICATIONS OF SHAOLIN CHIN NA 2	T013/394
DEFEND YOURSELF 1—UNARMED	T010/343
DEFEND YOURSELF 2—KNIFE	T011/351
EMEI BAGUAZHANG 1	T017/280
EMEI BAGUAZHANG 2	T018/299
EMEI BAGUAZHANG 3	T019/302
EIGHT SIMPLE QIGONG EXERCISES FOR HEALTH 2ND ED.	T005/54X
ESSENCE OF TAIJI QIGONG	T006/238
MUGAI RYU	T050/467
NORTHERN SHAOLIN SWORD—SAN CAI JIAN & ITS APPLICATIONS	T035/051
NORTHERN SHAOLIN SWORD—KUN WU JIAN & ITS APPLICATIONS	T036/06X
NORTHERN SHAOLIN SWORD—QI MEN JIAN & ITS APPLICATIONS	T037/078
QIGONG: 15 MINUTES TO HEALTH	T042/140
SCIENTIFIC FOUNDATION OF CHINESE QIGONG—LECTURE	T029/590
SHAOLIN KUNG FU BASIC TRAINING - 1	T057/0045
SHAOLIN KUNG FU BASIC TRAINING - 2	T058/0053
SHAOLIN LONG FIST KUNG FU—LIEN BU CHUAN	T002/19X
SHAOLIN LONG FIST KUNG FU—GUNG LI CHUAN	T003/203
SHAOLIN LONG FIST KUNG FU—ER LU MAI FU	T014/256
SHAOLIN LONG FIST KUNG FU—SHI ZI TANG	T015/264
SHAOLIN LONG FIST KUNG FU—TWELVE TAN TUI	T043/159
SHAOLIN LONG FIST KUNG FU—XIAO HU YAN	T025/604
SHAOLIN WHITE CRANE GONG FU—BASIC TRAINING 1	T046/440
SHAOLIN WHITE CRANE GONG FU— BASIC TRAINING 2	T049/459
SIMPLIFIED TAI CHI CHUAN—24 & 48	T021/329
SUN STYLE TAIJIQUAN	T022/469
TAI CHI CHUAN & APPLICATIONS—24 & 48	T024/485
TAIJI BALL QIGONG - 1	T054/475
TAIJI BALL QIGONG - 2	T057/483
TAIJI BALL QIGONG - 3	T062/0096
TAIJI BALL QIGONG - 4 MARTIAL APPLICATIONS	T063/010X
TAIJI CHIN NA	T016/408
TAIJI PUSHING HANDS - 1	T055/505
TAIJI PUSHING HANDS - 2	T058/513
TAIJI PUSHING HANDS - 3	T064/0134
TAIJI PUSHING HANDS - 4	T065/0142
TAIJI PUSHING HANDS - 5	T066/0150
TAIJI SABER	T053/491
TAIJI & SHAOLIN STAFF - FUNDAMENTAL TRAINING - 1	T061/0088
TAIJI SWORD, CLASSICAL YANG STYLE	T031/817
TAIJI YIN & YANG SYMBOL STICKING HANDS—YANG TAIJI TRAINING	T056/580
TAIJI YIN & YANG SYMBOL STICKING HANDS—YIN TAIJI TRAINING	T067/0177
TAIJIQUAN, CLASSICAL YANG STYLE	T030/752
WHITE CRANE HARD QIGONG	T026/612
WHITE CRANE SOFT QIGONG	T027/620
WILD GOOSE QIGONG	T032/949
WU STYLE TAIJIQUAN	T023/477
XINGYIQUAN—12 ANIMAL FORM	T020/310
YANG STYLE TAI CHI CHUAN	T001/181

COMPLETE DVDS FROM YMAA

ANALYSIS OF SHAOLIN CHIN NA (DVD)	DVD012/0231
CHIN NA INDEPTH COURSES 1 - 4 (DVD)	DVD001/602
CHIN NA INDEPTH COURSES 5 - 8 (DVD)	DVD004/610
CHIN NA INDEPTH COURSES 9 - 12 (DVD)	DVD005/629
EIGHT SIMPLE QIGONG EXERCISES FOR HEALTH (DVD)	DVD008/0037
ESSENCE OF TAIJI QIGONG (DVD)	DVD010/0215
SHAOLIN KUNG FU FUNDAMENTAL TRAINING - 1&2 (DVD)	DVD009/0207
SHAOLIN LONG FIST KUNG FU - BASIC SEQUENCES (DVD)	DVD007/661
SHAOLIN WHITE CRANE GONG FU BASIC TRAINING 1 & 2	DVD006/599
TAIJIQUAN CLASSICAL YANG STYLE (DVD)	DVD002/645
TAIJI SWORD, CLASSICAL YANG STYLE (DVD)	DVD011/0223
WHITE CRANE HARD & SOFT QIGONG (DVD)	DVD003/637

more products available from...

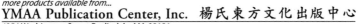

YMAA Publication Center, Inc. 楊氏東方文化出版中心

4354 Washington Street Roslindale, MA 02131
1-800-669-8892 • ymaa@aol.com • www.ymaa.com